The memoir received great reviews from book reviewers

Manhattan Book Review's Jennifer Padgett, who gave the book 4.5 stars out of 5, wrote "She (Mackall) writes with candor, simplicity, and authenticity about a subject that deserves attention… Her words exude courage, determination, and optimism…"

Maria Hughes of *The US Review of Books* named the memoir "a poignant read that summons the soul to drink deeper of life and not to sleep-walk through it." She wrote "Mackall's entries, however, are not meant to be just a glimpse into her mind. She seeks neither pity nor sympathy. Rather, she uses these experiences to be a clarion call to the reader."

San Francisco Book Review's Rachel Dehning called Mackall "an excellent example of a motivational speaker, constantly reminding people to savor the small things in life—the sunshine, the smells, and sights of nature—to really grasp what is important in life to help you to calm yourself."

Arron Washington of *Pacific Book Review* commends the book for teaching readers "about embracing life the way it is, taking care of ourselves, showing optimism and having a positive attitude during bad days, and moving on when terrible things happen to us."

"Telling her story not only creates awareness but also gives us an insight as to what cancer patients go through," said Washington in his review.

Susan Miller of *Seattle Book Review* found the book to be "an honest, heartfelt, and well-written book" and said the book made her "believe even more strongly in the importance of the here and now."

Tulsa Book Review's Kristi Elizabeth, who gave it all five stars, said she "really enjoyed this book because it was a true-life story that the author was brave enough to share and publish," commenting "It was very therapeutic."

Dying To Live Your Life

Dying To Live Your Life
Why does it take facing death to live your best life?

Lisabeth Mackall

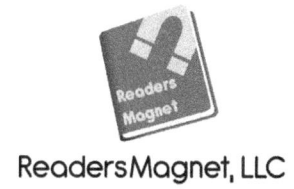

ReadersMagnet, LLC

Dying To Live Your Life: Why does it take facing death to live your best life?
Copyright © 2019 by Lisabeth Mackall

Published in the United States of America
ISBN Paperback: 978-1-949981-17-9
ISBN eBook: 978-1-949981-18-6

All rights reserved. No part of this publication may be reproduced, stored in a retrieval system or transmitted in any way by any means, electronic, mechanical, photocopy, recording or otherwise without the prior permission of the author except as provided by USA copyright law.

The opinions expressed by the author are not necessarily those of ReadersMagnet, LLC.

ReadersMagnet, LLC
10620 Treena Street, Suite 230 | San Diego, California, 92131 USA
1.619. 354. 2643 | www.readersmagnet.com

Book design copyright © 2019 by ReadersMagnet, LLC. All rights reserved.
Cover design by Ericka Walker
Interior design by Shemaryl Evans
Front cover photo credit by Ryan Mackall

Welcome to the journey of a lifetime. This journey, one that I did not want to take yet was forced to follow, delivers enlightenment like no other. Wisdom often follows traumatic experiences, but my wonder, on the backside of this adventure, is why does it take a trauma, a near death experience, for us to see the light? To find ourselves—to understand that we have a purpose far greater and deeper than the one that we are currently following.

I am a firm believer that if an individual can find the path that will lead them to living their best life, without the trauma that can trigger inner focus and enhanced listening to the world around them, then that person will be able to avoid the baggage of an injury to the soul.

I hope that the window into this life experience brings you to a new place in your own life—to find a way to begin your life anew. Each chapter is a walk through another month of life, of moments, another part of life that made an impact.

Before this story begins, another trying and scary life journey was documented in a book titled 27 Miles: The Tank's Journey Home. In that story begins the breaking down and building up of a wife, mother and individual that was the beginning of this new story.

Welcome to two years my life—two years of learning about life and death. Fear and Safety.

Learning how to see the real life that I was meant to live—month by month.

A life that you can learn as well.

One that only requires us to pay attention.

Contents

Chapter One
In the beginning... 13
Once Upon a Time 14
And so it begins 15
Remembering this moment 16
Waiting 17
The Hardest Part 18
The true journey starts tomorrow 20

Chapter Two
I should know better by now 23
Let the healing begin 25
What Does One Wear to the First Day of Chemo? 27
So how does it feel? 29
Chemo Day Two 31
Day Three post chemo 33

Chapter Three
The Power of Poop 36
WHERE I AM 40
Chemo Day Round Two 43

Chapter Four
Return from the tunnel 46
Life's Moments 48
Sunshine is the ultimate healer 51
The rules changed 53

Chapter Five
My nerves are showing 57
Going to Ground 59
Good news, good news, not so good news 61

Chapter Six
Ready, Set. 65
I'm just fine 67
Choices 69
Genetics, wounds and eyelashes 72
Another connected 74

Chapter Seven
Slowing things down 76
The Real Deal 78
Feeling the fatigue 79
Time and Priorities 81
It's just too much sometimes 83
One more down 85
Just a moment 86
Fun times 87

Chapter Eight
Keep on going 90
One foot in front of the other 92
Blessings in Four 93
Reality and Realization 96
It's Over 98
Short and sweet 99
Breathing a little easier 100

Chapter Nine
100% vs 50% 103
Community 105
Time to Rest 107
Time 109

Chapter Ten
Pain and Recovery 111
Bored is better than Pain 113
Perspective 2.0 114
Water journal 116

Chapter Eleven
Two weeks ago 120
Another day here 123
The Fear of Silence 124

Chapter Twelve
Limits vs Strength 128
Marching on 130
Pain–The Ultimate Equalizer 132
Good day Bad day 134

Chapter Thirteen
Please don't worry 136
Short update 138
I am Free 139
Witness for the New Year and an Anniversary 141
Finding Balance–Again 145
Carrying Wood 146
The Things I didn't know 148

Chapter Fourteen
What's new? 150
I Quit 153
A letter to my best friend 155
It's just Cancer 158
I love having cancer 160
Sitting in the dark 161
Figuring it out 162

Chapter Fifteen

This thing called lymphedema 164
27 Dresses–The Cancer version 166
It will be okay 168
So far so good 169
Moving on–Part 6 170
Boobs 2.0 172
Can't stop now 173
Impatient 174

Chapter Sixteen

Thinking about tomorrow 176
Moving on 177
More of the good 178
Happy One Year 179
Missed it 180
Only posting the good 181

Chapter Seventeen

The next big thing 183
Truth 185
Pain–1 Lisa–0 187
Pain–1 Lisa–1 188
New twist 189

Chapter Eighteen

My reality vs real reality 192
Beginning again 194
A few minutes alone 196
Thinking about it all 198
Not worrying about worrying 201
The "Eve" of things 203
I'm lucky 204

Chapter One

In the beginning...

At the start of any new life path, there is always a beginning, an event, or something, that marks the initiation into something new. As I began this book, my catalyst was cancer. A terrible diagnoses that continues to plague those around me—friends and colleagues, family members and acquaintances—and one that is all too familiar to all of us.

Cancer does not need to be the start of your own journey.

Your journey to a new life path, a new way to see the world and for the world to see you, can come within you.

You can choose to make your own start.

It takes a choice to be different, to be better.

And it takes guidance.

I hope that as you walk through the real time of change and enlightenment for me, that you can find your own mark, your own start, that brings you change.

Life is meant to be lived differently than most of us have been—living it coasting through and not seeing the amazing joy and beauty around us, within us, is a wasted life.

Don't waste the minutes that you have left by not noticing…

Once Upon a Time

March 4

Once upon a time a wife went to CaringBridge to tell the world about her husband. See, he was a police officer and had crashed his squad car, and almost died.

But this brave warrior didn't die, instead he fought back from his brain injury to return home to his family, and kept working hard to return to his family in blue.

But alas, he could not return. His wife, saddened by his despair, stayed by his side, loving him and encouraging him to find a new life.

And they did. Life moved on. New jobs, graduating children, new house. The sun began to shine again.

Until one day the wife was told some terrible news.

Breast cancer.

That can't be? Haven't we fought enough? Aren't we done fighting the hardest of battles?

Apparently not.

The wife, finding a love of writing in her new life, decides to step back into the world of sharing, and to the fondness she found in the purity of writing and the clarity of thought

Seeking hope, purging emotion, and praying for healing.

Do we start with the why me yet? Do I hit the road in despair? Start to drink?

I just don't know–time to pull on the big girl panties and figure this shit out.

And so it begins

March 6

Tomorrow at 0800 I meet with the first of what I presume will be many doctors. I am still residing in the world of disbelief, but I know that will quickly change to fight mode.

I have tried to not let any one thing in my life define me, and I am certainly not going to start now–this diagnosis will not own me.

I am grateful to those few souls that are in the know–quiet building of my close friends that I will need in the near future to help manage the load that I carry. I did learn the lesson following Frank's crash that no one can go alone, and if the fight I am facing is anything like the one that I fear is coming, it's going to take a village to carry us through this.

Two days ago I told a colleague about my news–she looked at me and asked "How resilient does someone have to be to be able to react as you are?"

I guess as resilient as it takes.

It's a word I have heard a lot the last three days since this diagnosis. To me it means we will figure this out as we go–right now, what I know is almost nothing.

Fear factor at its best.

Remember that show? People eating bugs, swimming naked with sharks, all for money and the title of winner? Right now I would be happy to eat some bugs to avoid what I fear will be another life altering, fear inducing stretch of time.

I have no idea if I will ever make this live. Right now it helps me to talk to myself–writing is cathartic for me. I will be able to look back and see the hope and positivity on days when I am feeling low.

It helped before and I truly hope it will help now.

Remembering this moment

March 8

The power of self-talk

Lisa–Remember today, remember yesterday. You are positive, grateful in fact, for the information that has been brought to you. Hearing that there is a tumor near the lymph node is a good thing, and can possibly mean that we are truly dealing with breast cancer, and not something bigger and scarier.

Remember how relieved you felt in that moment, remember the smile, and being thankful for that.

Today is a PET scan, and people are praying for good news. Cancer nowhere else means you tackle this with a vengeance, with everything you have, so that life can continue with hope.

Whatever the result, you have the power to face this with the strength and dignity that YOU want to bring to it.

Remember the saying "It is how you respond to the changes in life that make you who you are.

Remember the joy of now, the peace and comfort of the calm.

It will be okay

Love–Your heart

Waiting

March 9

The waiting is what is getting me today–waiting for the PET scan results, praying that it is good news, so we can move on in this process, and not dwell on what is. Either way the focus should be to look forward, but the fork in the road path is a big one.

One treatable, curable

The other, treatable.

I still have more questions than answers, and knowing that information out in the world contradicts itself makes decision making difficult.

Praying for news soon.

It's time to get this game started. The game I plan on winning.

The Hardest Part

March 9

Today was harder than any day in the 5 days that I have known I had breast cancer. Today was the day that I had to come to my children, again, and give them news that one of their parents was hurt. Telling my daughter was physically painful–we are so close, and united in so many ways–and I knew that she would be filled with fear. At 19, she is super smart, and will know the risk, and I can't protect her from that. As we talked she turned to me with tears running down her face and informed me that her semester paper and research is on breast cancer and optimism.

Coincidence? Probably not.

We waited until later in the evening to sit with the two younger boys. Of course, I looked at them and flashed back to that exact moment when I had to tell them that Frank, their Dad, was in the hospital, and wouldn't be coming home for a long time. Instead, I had to look them in the face and tell them that now it was me that was hurt. No parent should ever have to do that once, let alone twice. It just sucks.

AJ, my middle son, asked a lot of questions. Tommy, our youngest, put his head in his sisters' lap and cried, soon leaving the room in tears.

Next was a call to Ryan, the oldest boy, away at school, and of all, he fed back to me what I give to others–he listened, he told me he isn't worried because he knows I've got this, and that was it. Now that is a brave kid.

I have lots of "other" kids in my world, kids that grew up in our house or became surrogates along the way.

They too will be sad, and I hate that part for them.

I am not in pain for myself, but for those around me. I never want to hurt others or make them upset, and with each passing day more and more people know, and more and more people face me with tears. That hurts my heart more than I will ever let cancer hurt me.

Tomorrow I have to tell my work teams–some will cry, all will be shocked, and it will be another day of feeling good, but knowing the fight is coming.

This is a fight I refuse to lose–this is a fight that must be won.

Writing this out loud will be my savior–being able to talk to myself, purge out worry, and go to bed is awfully nice.

And I wonder if I have any words left in me for this fight–only time will tell.

The true journey starts tomorrow

March 10

Today was another day of tests and work. My goal for the day was to finish a large project at work, to communicate to the bulk of my team that life was going to change for me quickly, and in the midst of the day, squeeze in an echocardiogram and a chemo class. Fun times my friends, fun times.

I find that telling people that I have breast cancer hurts my heart–not for me, but for them. The people I surround myself with are kind, hard-working, engaged people. They care for others, they do for others–I wouldn't be around people that did not want to do the right thing, and work for the greater good. It is hard to tell people something like "I have breast cancer" but sometimes there is just no way around it.

I had to do it over and over again today. In truth, there were at least 15 times that I had to drop on someone "Hey, I need to tell you something." Being the introvert that I am, this level of heightened stressful communication is exhausting. It isn't that I am not positive and still feeling okay, it is just repeatedly feeling like I hurt people makes me feel bad.

I am grateful that my work team now knows–I had so many people check in today and tell me their own stories, pray over me, and just give me a hug.

Those moments I cherish each time they occur.

My main focus of tonight was to ensure that I reached out to as many people as possible before I begin informing people on social media–that and being available for the kids. Our children are so resilient. I just wish they did not have to absorb so much hardness in their lives. There were definitely more questions today, and worry statements and a lot of hugs. I hope that the more they see life is still the same, rules are still the same, and hopefully Mom still is the same, we can keep life together on some level.

On some levels I have no idea how this is going to go.

My prayer for tonight is to get through tomorrow–I worry about port placement–I just don't like things in my body.

I am pretty sure I have to get over that part. It is going to be part of my life for the next 5 months.

In just one week my life took an incredible turn, one that I could not imagine.

Moving from a regular "normal" life, to a life filled with doctors, nurses and needles can obliterate even the most solid, comfortable individual. Can anyone, even those grounded in their faith, face so much transition and change in such a short amount of time without rocking the core of who they are and what they believe?

How does one see and find a future not knowing what each day will bring?

We are not in control of so much around us, and when we give that up, and just BE in our days, life suddenly changes. Allowing the life that is lived to be noticed, from the smallest to the biggest things in a day, brings a new level of harmony to the life that you live.

For me during this first week of cancer life, I lived on the facts. I ate them for breakfast, snacked on them in the afternoon, and digested them at night.

I wanted as many of them as I could find, so that I could control them.

They built up walls of strength around me, so that I felt that none of the bad stuff could come in. I was going to control the destiny of what would happen to me with the facts.

But the facts could not protect me from the assault of treatment.

And facts can remove us from noticing the things around us that are there to engage us, even in the hard and scary moments.

For anyone starting something catastrophically new–a death, new unpredictable changes, loss, or heartbreak–reality seems to take a back seat. It is hard to believe what is happening, how quickly things can change, and I can remember the days of denial.

Thinking that it really can't be all THAT bad can it? This can't be terminal cancer, or the treatment really won't be a big deal.

How could that happen to me? To us?

The truth is anything can happen to anyone. I am a firm believer that because we are all humans, anything that a human is subject to can invade a life. It doesn't matter if you are rich and living in a mansion, or living paycheck to paycheck, life intervenes.

And when it does, you have a decision to make.

You either live life, for whatever moments you have left, or you let whatever is happening, take over.

But you get to choose—you choose where you put your energy. You choose the path you will take.

Even if other things get in the way, like chemo, pain or money, you still get to choose your reactions to those things.

And the choices are what make each moment.

There is a big difference between knowing what is going on around you, and SEEING and FEELING what is going on around you. When you learn that lesson, life will never be the same. Life will always hold wonder. Amazement. Even in the hard dark times.

It is a lesson that I did not learn for some time.

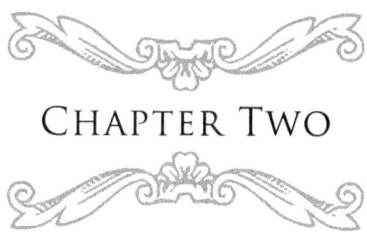

Chapter Two

I should know better by now

March 11

Today for me was the ultimate in scary—which turned into a funny great day.

For some reason, the thought of having a port placed under my skin, and knowing it will live there for the next 5 months freaked me out. I wanted no part of it at all.

My fear is unfounded, made large and in charge in my brain by not trusting in myself and those around me. I learned this lesson over and over in the last few years, and woke up this morning trying to recalibrate myself so I wouldn't freak out.

I woke up early, and decided some yoga would help calm the steel ball rolling around in my stomach. The funny part about yoga is that it also reminds me that I am 45 and not quite as flexible as I used to be. Breathing and stretching is absolutely the best medicine for me, and before I knew it, Frank and I were headed to the hospital. It was weird walking in as a patient instead of an employee, and lucky me, the minute I hit the Outpatient Unit, they were ready for me to go back.

I really was okay and calm until after my first few visits from the great nurses and the doc. It was that alone time that started to bring the panic back. I literally closed my eyes and just listened to myself breathe for a few minutes, and then my ride arrived.

Talking to people at least distracts me from thinking, especially as I wheeled towards the surgical suite. But then one of the few things that could help me in the world started to happen. The nurse that was with me, a good looking guy, started to give me a little bit of crap.

And to tell really bad jokes.

And then the other one started in with even worse jokes.

They told me if I was laughing that they would know that the meds were working. I quickly told them that I had not had enough meds, and then...

Nothing. It was over.

I woke up with Frank in my room and my comedian saviors gone.

I know that when I ask for peace and solace, it arrives. This time instead of my family from law enforcement, it was my hospital family, and they came through with flying colors.

I can only imagine how much fun things will be in chemo next week.

Ponies? Dancing monkeys? Strippers?

Only time will tell....

Thanks for all of your prayers today my friends.

Let the healing begin

March 14

I say that as I realized today that I am not waiting for chemotherapy to start my healing–I am already healing.

Being diagnosed with breast cancer makes you re-evaluate everything in your life, from what your priorities are, to what you eat every day. When I started assessing my life, I realized that it isn't going to be chemo that saves my life, it is going to be me that saves my life.

I have spent nine days looking at my life and what I will need in the next year fighting this battle. I know I need peace, I need calm.

I need to be relaxed and I need to be free from worry. I need good nutrition, sleep and information.

But most of all I am going to need help.

Now for me, that is the HARDEST thing for me to accept. I am the helper. I am the one that sends the help, brings the help, is the help.

But once, four years ago, I accepted the help.

And it is time for me to soon be in that place again.

Our world is, well, complicated. It isn't as easy as passing along the daily life from one person to another. There is a carefully constructed scaffolding that surrounds our life, and that delicate balance keeps all of us on an even keel.

I will be unable to keep that balance alone.

Right now is the time for me to shore up that balance. Careful organization and information gathering is the key to this success.

That, and the incredible people that revolve around us offering everything from food to childcare shuttling, cleaning and hanging out with me at chemo. We are so blessed, there are times when I cannot fathom how we became to reside on the receiving end of such an amazing supportive community. Although it is hard for me to accept that we will be on the receiving end of so much support again, there is part of my heart that is forever grateful that I know it is there.

Fear has no place in this journey, but that doesn't mean that it isn't hiding there in the shadows of my heart. It doesn't get to visit often, but occasionally it rears its ugly head into my space, and I have to give it a bit of attention.

I am not a Pollyanna, I know that this is not going to be easy. I understand that there are no guarantees in this journey, and that ultimately, I can only do my part.

The rest is not up to me.

For those medical people in my world that want tangible information, here you go. The hormone results were positive so I will go on hormone suppression therapy when we are through with all of this. My HER2 is negative. Now for me not to know how big a deal this was was amusing to me. Apparently, I really did not want to have to fight that as well. Treatment plan remains the same–chemo starts this Thursday. Lucky for me I get to work in the morning and then head downstairs for treatment (yes, yes I know, take it easy, I hear you).

I have chemo every other week for 8 weeks, then switch to every week for the next 12. After that we will see how things go. I am planning surgery in the future, but you never know where the journey may take us.

Thank you again for all of your kind words and support.

Somehow writing just makes things better.

What Does One Wear to the First Day of Chemo?

March 16

Silly, right? For me, I have thought about this quite a bit this afternoon, trying to figure out what to wear.

I am not great at the "girl" thing, preferring other people to tell me what looks good, and then me agreeing to wear it. I just don't like thinking about clothes. For me, clothes are the best when they involve sweatpants and a large comfy sweatshirt. That is bliss.

But for me tomorrow, my first day of the second weapon we are throwing at breast cancer, I am working. Why not? Why sit at home and think about your body being filled with a toxic substance that is going to kill cancer, and probably some other cells as well.

Why not go to work and be around people that will distract you, ask questions, get to work on a project or two, and THEN head downstairs to a room almost directly below my office, and begin the fun then.

For me, that is what works. And since I cannot wear sweatpants to work, I will have to figure something else out.

Over the last few days I have begun to imagine what I am sure countless of others have thought of before they started chemo.

Does it hurt going in? Do you feel it? Will I super vomit? Will it make me tired right away?

So many thoughts go through my head right now, although honestly they are more curious than fearful. I know there are risks, I know there is no guarantee, I know there is the good chance that I will not feel so hot.

But I also know that I feel positive, I feel good, and that I feel motivated to make this an experience that is not only tolerated, but one that I live through in a way that isn't devastating to me as a person. I think that many of us headed into chemo want to be sure that we don't lose ourselves in this process.

I think that maybe that is my biggest fear.

I don't want to lose myself in this process.

Fighting cancer sucks, but I don't want it to take over me.

I don't want it to define my every day, my every moment–my entire life.

My goal is to have many moments that I feel like myself–maybe not my usual 100% full of energy self–but myself. I am still going to be me.

Maybe a me without my red hair, a me without my usual never-ending energy, a me that cannot keep 26 balls in the air juggling at once.

But me, I just want to be me.

I will let you know how tomorrow how it goes, I am curious to see where this part of the journey takes me tomorrow.

So how does it feel?

March 17

I know you are dying to ask? How does it feel to have toxic chemicals pumped into your body, along with a mountain of drugs to prevent nausea?

Truly, it feels like nothing–right now.

I am sitting in the chemo chair, listening to music, and working. I thought I would take a break to make sure I write down this much anticipated (with worry) the first day of this process.

I was scared of the first punch to my port–I hear that it can be painful. I anticipated that and fretted more about that today than any other part of this process. My nurse was great and talked me through each part right up to the punch, and did a 1-2-3. Nothing.

That was it–I felt nothing.

And again I was reminded of the power of people, prayer and believing.

I asked for no pain, I meditated about not being in pain, and I prayed for no pain.

And no pain.

The drugs are moving in–the first drug is done, injected slowly by my nurse as we talked about the kids. It was bright red and I was warned that it will change the color of your urine–good thing they tell you that or THAT'S a surprise. My second drug is running now and other than beginning to feel like I am tired from stress, all is well.

I know the future of this will change, and I feel for all of these people sitting here with me today also getting chemo.

How many of us are here.

How rampant is cancer in our society.

How invasive are the things we eat, drink, clean with, and have in our homes every day.

It makes you wonder.

Sitting here getting chemo and thinking about every single thing I eat these days' makes you wonder what in my world contributed to this.

I know some of this is genetic, but it makes you wonder...

Chemo Day Two

March 19

It is interesting to try to reflect on the last 24 hours.

I spent my first day post chemo at work, feeling a little shaky, a little punky, and eventually headed downstairs for my follow up shot. My nurse is a wonderful kind soul who poked and prodded at me both physically and emotionally to ensure that I was doing okay on my first day post chemo.

Of course I insisted that I was fine, but did confess that I was not feeling too hot and I was a bit cold. She gave me the "face" (you know that face, the one your mother or a good friend will make), which meant that I needed to stop and think about what I needed at this moment. Although I had had a fine day, it was getting to the end and heading home started to sound really nice.

I packed up my stuff and realized as I was heading home how tired I was–tired enough that it was time for a nap.

Deciding that I needed to take the meds that would make me feel better, I did just that. The relief of snuggling into bed and letting go a little bit was heaven, and knowing that nothing else was needed at that moment was great. The kids and Frank had dinner, I got to rest and stay warm, and all was well with the evening.

Today, after a really good night's sleep, I headed off for my wig appointment. I was excited for this part of the journey, and felt I had chosen wisely for the where to go–a marathon runner who also was hit with breast cancer in her 40's.

She now owns a wig shop, and is amazing in her execution, energy and skills. With my heart sister and friend Kriscel by my side, we found exactly what I needed, which is different than what I thought I needed. A little longer than now, a little shorter than before, it meets in the middle of where life was and is–the perfect place.

So today's picture is of the now hair, the hair that I have for the next few weeks, and then it will change again.

That's fine with me, change is coming anyway. Can't stop it.

Today's plan is rest–energy conservation has become my new planning friend.

Rest it is. Oh, and eating.

Not my favorite thing right now but not an option. My diet is so different that sometimes it is hard to make sure I am eating enough.

Time for some peanut butter toast.

Day Three post chemo

March 20

So I am holding on to my day three, which for me means that this should be the last day of feeling like I have the flu.

That is my plan anyway, but as we all know, life does not go according to my plan. Clearly, since none of this was on my agenda.

Yesterday I learned a lesson in energy conservation–that what I think is conservation may not be what my body feels is conservation. Even though I spent the day resting, taking out our son for his belated birthday dinner was all I did, and I was done before dinner was finished.

No soccer, no end of night clean up, just bed.

It is not like you can fight it, the more you fight it the worse you feel, and that's not okay. So off to bed I went, in my head complaining the whole time.

I don't like not having control of my usually fit and functional self.

I have decided to not work out or do yoga on the first three days post–chemo–guided imagery and diet will be the focus, along with lots of rest. After that we will see if we can get back to walking and light exercise so I can stay on some track of healthy during all of this.

I am overwhelmed with the offers to help us–yes, food delivery is getting organized, yes, people are working on other things as well. All I can say is that it is hard to accept as always. Saying yes is hard.

I am trying.

Time to add more food to my very controlled diet–no sugar was much easier than I thought it would–I guess when your life is on the line you will be happy to give up anything to ensure that you will be here for a long time.

Sugar and chocolate are a drop in the bucket.

When one begins the day, any day, thinking that it will be one thing, and then transitions into something completely different, you can usually handle the change. Life often does that, makes a sharp right turn when you were sure you were going to head left.

When life drops an unexpected bombshell into your life, it creates a crater no different than a meteor hitting earth. In that one second, everything changes. You are no longer the same person that you were just a day ago, an hour ago, or even a few minutes ago.

I remember how heightened my senses seemed to be at some of those specific moments—what the ceiling tiles looked like in the surgery suite, the smell of the hand foam in the hospital, and even the frame on the painting in the chemo room.

Snapshots of life become more vivid than before—and these snapshots can be good or not so good.

It comes early on in this process of change—at least in hindsight—that if I could just control everything around me, I would continue to be okay.

If I could control what happens to my hair, it will be okay.

If I can control the pain, it will be okay.

If I can control the chemo, it will be okay.

Nowhere in any of this did I begin to realize that I do not control anything in this process. I may THINK that I have control, but truly, am I running this show?

In my head, I sure thought I did.

But control, or the illusion of control, is not fact.

It is a fairy tale.

The only control that is truly within us is how we react to the world around us. If you reread my daily writings, controlling things around me made me feel better. It made me feel like I was doing "something" to make sure that I would be okay, whatever okay meant at that time.

Instead of trying to control everything around me, would I have been better served by just "being" in those moments? By paying attention to the nurses helping me, or the beautiful painting in the chemo room, could I have made the moment less worrisome by being more engaged in the moments?

Maybe. Probably.

Appreciation and noticing the things that are good, even in the tough moments, can bring a completely different perspective.

Even in the exact moment that toxic chemo drugs began to flow through my IV, was there something that in that moment would have made me smile? Made me grateful, feel purposeful, or even brought me joy?

It is hard to imagine that I could have had those thoughts in that moment, but I believe that it is possible to find greatness there.

It is about perspective.

And how we look at the world.

In those moments, I was just not quite ready to see what was around me. I wanted to control what I felt, what I paid attention to, and how I reacted to everything. To be honest, as I write those words, I realize the ridiculousness of that, but while in the moment, anyone would try to make sure they were okay.

What is the other option? Falling apart? Crying, screaming and losing complete control?

How would that help this situation? Things are going to happen whether or not I approve, control or think about this process. What I should have done, and I what I chose to do during these days, are two very different things.

I chose control, joking, working and a strong focus on not feeling—plowing through the days, feigning "okayness" and not giving in to the situation.

If I had stepped back, just for a moment, and realized that it would have been okay to be sad, scared and maybe even wonder how it would be to let go, even for just a little bit, would it have made my life different at that time?

I believe it would have…

Right now, in your own moment, can you see what is around you?

Chapter Three

The Power of Poop

March 23

Yep–you see that right. And I know you are thinking "this is going to be TMI, more than I want to know, and probably not something that I want to read."

Well then, my thought is, that's okay, don't read it :) I am trying to walk myself through this process, and sometimes the truth is uncomfortable.

The last few days have been pretty rough–I know, chemo and all, but I really wanted to have my three days and then head back to my life in between these "disruptions" to my normal life.

I did not want this to take over; I did not want this to become me.

So Monday morning I kept trying to convince myself that I was better. That I felt good.

But I didn't. I kinda felt lousy.

I blamed it on some of the meds that I am taking to try and keep me from puking–important stuff. But I still didn't feel good. I checked all of the paperwork to read up on symptoms, and thought that maybe I needed to eat more to settle my stomach and get rid of these yucky feelings. Food didn't help, and by mid-afternoon, it was time to go home and take a nap. I still had time with the kids, and time with Frank, but it certainly was not a great night.

The next day I thought "okay this will be better." But another morning was met with yucky stomach and real light-headedness. A call into the cancer center and I had what I thought was an answer to what ailed me–water.

The question posed to me was simple–are you peeing every hour? The answer was a resounding no. I wasn't.

So I was probably dehydrated! Well that is easy to fix–water, more water, some tea and some water. And then the peeing. ALL. THE. TIME.–12 huge glasses of fluid later I knew that I was no longer dehydrated.

But at least I should feel better now.

I woke to high hopes this morning of being done, being back to myself.

Nope. Felt like crap. Again. And I am starting to worry.

Is this how this is really going to go? I am not going to get ANY break in this process at all? I am going to feel fuzzy, ill, and miserable for the next 5 months! I just can't.

And to be honest, it was the first time that I was scared.

I made it to work, but not without having to sit in the parking ramp waiting area on the floor so I didn't pass out in the elevator.

I got to my office, and sat still.

This was real. This is how it feels, and I am not sure that I can do this.

And I started to tear up.

I am blessed with smart and timely workmates–and one stopped me in the kitchen and asked how I was feeling.

My response was "eh" and was met with concern. We started to talk out how I was feeling, and as we chatted, I realized what I may have done.

How many glasses of water is too many? Hmmm, apparently it is 12.

I had essentially wiped out the minerals and salt in my system and put myself into electrolyte imbalance- highly unpleasant.

Behold the power of Gatorade. And with that slight change I felt life slowly start to return to normal. Throughout the day multiple Gatorades put me back into line–but not all was right with the world.

Although I finally started to feel better, my stomach.... oh the stomach.

Now I am not going to gross you out with details, but let's just say that things were not moving, and as I calculated, had not for days.

Days and days.

Now, our bodies are marvelous machines–food and liquids go in, and the "waste" goes out. Our bodies process everything that we put into it, the good and the bad. Sometimes that system does not work well, and when it doesn't it can certainly upset the balance.

Now with my system, being pumped full of toxic chemicals to kill the cancer, my system is highly overloaded with toxins. I am asking a lot of my body–to process and use the nutrition I put into it to kill and repair cancer cells, and to help build and hold together my good cells to fight back.

My body is working at 150% to help me out, and I realized that I may not be paying enough attention.

In all this work, my body processes are not reacting like they always have–systems are changing, reacting to this treatment, and what I expect to happen is not happening. So instead of purging all of these toxins, I have been holding on to them.

And holding, and holding. You get the picture.

Lucky for me, the electrolyte "rebalance" and the purge of the system has had a miraculous change in my overall happiness with the universe. Although not fully returned to normal, it is clear that a body does not work well, when it is not working well.

What I have to remember is that my body is different now, and I need to work with it and not against it. My wise medical director told me today that I don't have my normal body awareness anymore–what has worked and happened for 45 years isn't happening anymore and I have new rules, of which no one has handed me the playbook.

I have to pay attention, and try to find the delicate balance that is my system now, so that it can work for me.

Lessons learned, balance restored, and although I may not be back to all of "me" tomorrow, at least I have learned a new lesson on this journey.

You can follow the rules, think you are doing what is right, but all bets are off, and it is important to try and find the "balance."

WHERE I AM

March 28

I realized today that it has been many days since I wrote anything. In my head that is a funny statement, since I write blog posts all the time, talking to myself throughout the day. However, it has become difficult to ensure that they actually make it here at the end of the day.

I am grateful that life settled down and return to a more typical pattern following the "great stomach fiasco" of Chemo Round One. As I look back, I realized how over-focused I had become on the big picture, and how little I was paying attention to what my body was telling me. I understand that part of that process is learning; no one really knows how they will react to chemo, but I also know some pretty basic things about nutrition, hydration and recovery that apparently went completely out the window last week.

Lucky for me, I get to try and successfully navigate this path again starting this Thursday when I enter the ring again for Chemo Round Two. My hopes for this time around are that I,

1. Remember to eat, drink and take my meds, and: 2. Have a better outcome following my magical three day window.

I know I am not guaranteed any of those things, but I do hope that I can take advantage of what I have learned and put it to good use.

Sometimes when I walk through the hospital, I see people that I have not run into in the last few weeks. Most of them immediately comment on my short hair, especially knowing how long it was before. Because I am me, I tell them that I did it because I wanted to see how it looked before it fell out, and I tell them about my diagnoses.

I forget how scary the words BREAST CANCER are–how when I googled my original diagnosis, how my heart dropped out of my chest. I saw that look today when I had to tell one of my colleagues why I cut my hair, and the shock and tears were enough for me to pause in my head.

I think that I have become somewhat immune to the fear factor, because I have accepted that this is what I have, that my battle plan is in place, and that I am certain of success.

But those words–breast cancer–are scary to most people.

After I shocked my friend, and moved on to my later meetings in the day, I thought about how I communicate this to people, and if I am doing the right thing by being so matter-of-fact about the situation. Truly, I am not sure I can be any other way, this is who I am, but it did give me pause to wonder if I need to temper my delivery.

Breast cancer sucks; that is a true fact.

Having a mountain of tests performed to further solidify the diagnosis, being poked and prodded, and having surgeries to prepare for chemo and radiation is not pleasant.

Sitting in a room waiting for that first round of chemo really sucks. But the truth is, it is still here. I still have it. Others still have it. And we have to figure out to live while we have it.

I think that is why I am so factual with my delivery.

I have breast cancer.

Once said, then I can move on in the day. I still am me, I am just me with breast cancer.

This week will be an interesting transition week for me–I am supposed to lose my hair sometime in the very near future, and I am feeling "something" about that, although I cannot pinpoint what that feeling is. I am fine with the hair loss, I don't like it, but it won't be that big a deal.

However, I realized today that I miss my hair. I played with it a lot, and as Frank said, "you are not quite you without the red hair." I think that is what I am feeling right now. I have a wig, and I think

I might wear it, but I am not so sure about that either. I need to decide who I am wearing it for, and why.

Right now I see many others in the waiting area, further along than me, wearing their cute hats, looking tired, and I think "well, there it is, I will be there soon."

But I am not sure I want to be there. I am not sure I want to wear a hat.

Because am I not still me without the red hair?

That is part of my internal struggle right now—will I still be Red to my law enforcement family?

(Two minute pause)

Well, since I always work from a place of complete honesty, I get to now post that writing that last sentence made me burst into tears. Yuck, crying sucks almost as bad as breast cancer.

But honesty of emotion is what carried me through the last journal pathway so no need to change that cycle now.

Clearly it means more than I think it does—and the redhead in me is heartbroken.

Chemo Day Round Two

March 31

So as with the last time, chemo day was relatively uneventful.

The process is systematic and planned out, and I returned to work to finish up my day. I came home and organized kids, dinner, taxes and then decided enough was enough. The feelings of the first few hours are difficult to explain–I tried at work and the best description is that I feel like I am full. Knowing how much fluid they run into me during this process it is not surprising that I feel this way. Usually it goes away fairly quickly, but tonight it is lingering and giving me a headache.

Eventually it will let go and I will get some sleep. For now, it feels yucky. Yep, that is the clinical and technical word I am going to stick with right now.

My prayers are that this process follows a similar pattern as the last one, without the self-created issues that I made for myself the last time. I have a conference presentation on Saturday and hoping that we can make it through that without incident. I have built in lots of rest, quiet and breaks.

And yes I will take my meds–I know what you are thinking.

The journey is not an easy one–there are days like today and the next few which try your patience as a breast cancer fighter. I long for the easy days, when you can "forget" that you are dealing with cancer. It comes back into hard focus when you are actually engaged in a fight with your body.

Off to rest.

Doctors orders.

One month of my life had gone by.

In that time, I would normally not even pause to think about what I have done in that month, where I have been, or what I may have missed.

Most often I am always looking ahead, to the next thing, the next soccer game, meeting, appointment or schedule that is coming up next.

I don't dwell or linger, I don't stick or get stuck.

But maybe I need to learn to savor things a bit more.

That month changed me—it would change anyone, how can it not? Your body is being changed with poison that should cure you of a disease that changed who you feel that you are.

Life has changed in that you spend so much time with doctors and nurses that you didn't even know a month ago, and now they know you by name.

And by diagnosis.

A month after cancer diagnosis is a month of intense change, often whipping by us without any option of slowing things down to notice anything. I definitely noticed the things happening to my body—hard to not focus on pending hair loss, stomach issues, eating differently, being tired all the time. But did I noticed anything else? Was I even aware of the other things going on in my life, around my life, or is it too difficult to step away from what is happening to me, to notice the things happening around me?

We all know the saying that change is a constant.

Change is fine in my book, and truly, I like to change things around sometimes just to keep life interesting. But change brought on by cancer, treatment and fear, these are changes that I am not prepared for.

Sometimes I wish it would all slow down, just for a minute, so I would notice the snow fall, listen to the wind in the trees outside my windows, smell the candle burning in the kitchen, or listen to the music playing in the atrium.

But I was wrapped up in myself, my fear, my internal struggle with what was happening to me. I wanted to notice more, to see more around me, but I was not ready. I was not present enough in a way that allowed me to pause.

I will learn the skill of the pause. Of the deep breathe.

In. And out.

In. And out.

Think of breathing in a large balloon that can only be emptied by slowly pushing it from the back. The art of breathing is the first lesson in learning to slow down. Breathing apps, articles and programs are available on every electronic device, and I recommend you seek them out. When I finally learned to breathe, and relearned, and learned again (and am STILL learning) life changed for me.

Breathing is part of life—it is essential.

And when we focus on breathing, all of a sudden you notice other things.

It is the beginning of a new beginning of awareness.

Chapter Four

Return from the tunnel

April 5

Have you ever been on a trip that you did not want to go on? That trip that you know has an end, but also has a beginning that cannot be avoided?

I am returning back from that trip again, the trip that I still have to make two more times—and a small piece of me is starting to protest.

I am starting to figure out the process, my reactions, and my responses to each of these journeys. As I come off the second round of four for this drug, I have learned more, but I have also realized that there is a true toll to be paid each and every time I follow this path—a toll hit to my very soul that I have to decide how to handle.

Every other Thursday I get to board a train that is going to travel to a darker place, into a mountain tunnel lit only by the train's single powerful headlight. The rails are straight and the journey into the mountain is the only way to get to the other side. Each day following treatment brings you deeper into the mountain, each moment moving you forward even in the times when you don't feel like moving forward. The days click ahead, until you realize that the darkness and fuzziness are slowly receding, and the light, just ahead, has appeared again, just like you knew it would.

Now those that saw me this weekend, or at work the last few days would not guess that this is what it feels like–and truly, for the most part, my journey through the mountain this time was not what I would call terrible. But as I sat in the bathtub tonight trying to warm up from my now" chronic-chilly due to baldness" I realized that a crack has formed in my steadfast resiliency.

I'm kind of sick of this already.

And I have a long way to go.

Now, tomorrow morning, if my pattern of recovery resumes, I will wake up feeling pretty darn good, almost back to normal, and can resume my fast paced life. But a small part of me tonight is already dreading the next time, and the subsequent path that has to be taken to recover.

It is unusual for me to allow myself time to fret about things that I cannot control. When things are going to happen that I cannot change, I look at them with a clear conscious, a critical eye, and try to find the path that makes the most sense for me. This has held me true for many years, allowing me to work through many fears and concerns, especially the last four years.

I hold the belief that by nurturing the good parts of any moment, and there are always good parts, the harder pieces seem to fall by the wayside.

I know I am not going to walk through this process unscathed–I am just a bit surprised at the niggle of worry that has entered into my sphere of thought this evening. It isn't a worry about my recovery, it is the understanding that next week I have to start things again, and I don't want to,

But guess what–I don't always get what I want.

Another week of feeling good will come, another week where I can return to my regularly scheduled life, interrupted by breast cancer.

I am thankful for the warmer breeze, the promise of Spring, the gardens that await.

They will tide me over in the times of the tunnel traveling, knowing that I will always come out on the other side.

Life's Moments

April 10

If you followed my journey with my husband, you know that I took to the heart the message that I believe God sent me, encouraging me to pay attention to the things in my life that are precious and important. That message was for me to encourage others to do the same.

Life is a fast-paced chaotic journey for so many of us, that amazing and beautiful moments fly by us without a second thought. It is simple to just keep going with the head down, phone checking, racing by attitude many of us have–why not? It gets us where we are going, although I can assure you, much is missed when the journey is lived that way.

Before BC (breast cancer) I would say that I had still retained much of that focused life philosophy, and tried to live it in a way that others might notice, and change their lives to pay attention. When you are given gifts of time and understanding in your life, I have always felt that it was then my job to pass that along. To tell others.

To share the story so that in the midst of the hurt and trauma, good can come from it.

That is what I am meant to do with my life.

I just was not aware that the plan was for me to do it again.

So in these days, I write. A lot. In my head.

Which I have found is not always effective since no one else is living up there but me. The new goal is to at least update 2-3 times a week, instead of one. Especially to write on the days that I feel well, as I know my writing is heavily colored by the level of toxins floating around in my system. That was wise advice from my good friend Elizabeth last night—ensuring that people know that I am mostly okay, with a side order of crappy on a few days each week.

I learned another lesson this past week and it was one that I am still struggling to accept in my head.

The conversation was around the fact that I am sick, and that I need help.

I do not accept either of those well, especially the sick part. I don't get sick.

It is something that I have been fairly blessed with throughout my life and through genetics or healthy eating, have stayed relatively "well" most of my life. Knowing I am labeled "extremely healthy, with metastatic breast cancer" has helped me to maintain that image in my head, instead of heading down the rabbit hole of being sick.

I accept that I have breast cancer, but saying I am sick? I do not accept that.

Knowing that there are times I will need help? Yes, but saying I need help because I am sick? No. Denied.

I have cancer, and that sucks.

But I have stated out loud, and written on the white board in my office, that this does not define me. I am not "Lisabeth Mackall, sick with breast cancer" I am "Lisabeth Mackall. I have a life.

And I have breast cancer."

The issue I have is with accepting that there are limitations to what I can do, and where my energy should be spent. I can do that.

The other issue is communicating with my family when I am unable to do my normal level of activity, without walking in the door knowing I need to go lie down, and exploding at everyone because nothing is done.

And why should it be when I always take care of things.

Sooooo, where does the blame lie on that?? That is with me, and being able to tell my family and those around me that "today, I need help with this." Today I need you to ....."

And that is on the far end of extremely difficult for me–but I am trying.

I just can't do it and use the words "because I am sick."

Our family therapist tried to help me frame that earlier in the week–and I struggled. I finally accepted that maybe I can communicate that CHEMO is making me feel crappy so then I need help.

I think I might be able to live with that.

Especially because chemo does make you feel crappy.

So for me, the challenge is two-fold: allowing others to help, and ensuring I am finding those moments of joy and fun every day.

Yesterday was one of those moments for me–driving home from our youngest boys birthday party, I had 5 teenage boys in the car. A song came on the radio and they ALL started singing at once. On top of that, each round was accented by the fun sounds made by a jar of fart putty.

Those my friends, are the moments that we need to pay attention to–priceless and ridiculous.

But oh so important.

Sunshine is the ultimate healer

April 14

So 3 down, 1 to go–that is what is in my head right now, although as I sit here, in a sun puddle in my living room, I know that today is not the day that is hard.

Today is a bit stressful, as there was some worry that I may not be able to do chemo today as my port site has a spot that isn't healing, and I have an infection. I ended up meeting with my doc and we talked about how I was feeling, my labs (all normal) and by the time we were done decided that chemo was a go. It put me behind a bit on the schedule, but eventually all of the multiple bags of fluid and toxic fun were loaded into my system, and I left feeling like I always do–like an overfilled balloon.

Every vein in my body bulging with fluid. It is so weird, hard to describe except maybe when you have a really bad sinus infection but you can breathe just fine.

I don't like it much.

We did chat today about my day 5 and 6, which are unpleasant. I am hoping to make them better–of course by the time I figure all of this out, this drug will be over and I will transition to the next phase of my chemo protocol, and have to figure out another drug.

Fun times.

Anyone that knows me knows that I crave sunshine and heat. When Frank and I were in Jamaica years ago, I wore sweats. And my bathing suit top, but sweats. I wanted to be hot, and I loved every minute of it. Some of my best years were living in Dallas, and stepping outside into that heat always brought me just a touch of joy, even on the hottest of days.

It recharges my soul.

I have been patiently waiting for the arrival of heat and sun. I have as part of my wellness plan time in the sun–both for the Vitamin D which I need for healing, and for the meditation and healing properties that my entire being gets from the sun. Gardening is a passion, and done best in the heat. I look forward to getting some gardening done this year at the new house, although I certainly will not be able to do what we had originally planned–I am sure I will not have that amount of energy.

But I will be outside.

If you are not a sun person, it is hard to explain the power that one can get from basking in the sunshine. For me, it is like drinking a cold glass of water when you are really hot–you get that first cold sip in your mouth, and you can already feel yourself refreshed, and with that first swallow, the coolness slips down your throat, each inch taking away the heat that you felt, bring coolness and energy back to you.

That is what the sun does for me. Closing my eyes, and feeling the sun heat on my face, I can feel each cell in my body expanding into new life, breathing deeper, absorbing energy, and creating new life within me. The sun for me is like my own personal healing well, and today my friends, I went back to the well.

When Frank and I left the hospital after chemo, we went to lunch. I immediately sat at a table bathed in sunshine, and after 15 minutes, Frank was so hot he had to move over to the shade. I smiled and was happy to move with him, as by then I was toasty. When we got home I immediately went outside and sat on the deck. I turned my face to the sky and breathed in deep.

This is EXACTLY what I need. This will help me pull through and I know that it will have a powerful impact over my next 6 days of chemo system purge. I am so grateful that there will be sun in my life for several of those days.

The fun part is trying to juggle the "I need Vitamin D so sit in the sun" with "this medication may cause sensitivity to sun and precaution should be taken when in direct sunlight."

Screw it. I vote for sun

The rules changed

April 18

I have often wondered if each of my chemo sessions would follow the same path each time. I was told that they may be similar in nature, and I have banked on that the last two sessions, and they have followed the same pattern. Well, this last round, round three, turned out to be an entirely different process.

Typically for me, the first three days after chemo have been not too bad for me to get through. I have worked, done presentations, carried on with my life, and then had some down days on the 5-6 days post my chemo sessions. I didn't like the down time, but I understood that sooner or later my life was going to be interrupted by my breast cancer, and the treatment that occurs. In fact, this time was not what I had planned, and it took me by surprise.

Instead of working all day Friday and getting through the weekend of soccer in Milwaukee, I spent most of the weekend lying low and feeling like just plain crap.

And I didn't like it at all.

I don't get sick, remember? I get a cold, or a down day, but this? What the hell is this?

It feels like a betrayal of my body, not doing what i want it to do, but truly, it isn't my body's fault, it is chemo's fault.

So today, I am regrouping, feeling a little bit better, and knowing that I could still have some rough days in the next few that were my typical "down days" but what a shift in dynamic for me.

Spending time with Frank is wonderful—we rarely have just quiet time together to chat, and sit still in the same space. We both agree that although I am not at my best by far, it is still nice to just be home together.

Chemo is not a kind part of life–it is a vicious drug that has a purpose, but getting through it is so hard. I am thankful that I appear to be coming out on the other side of this round, but slightly worried that my last round of this drug may hit me this hard again. Hard to know what to expect, but that is life anyway right?

No day has a guarantee–and that is true for all of us.

So this morning, I spent 20 minutes out front while Tommy made shots on his hockey net while waiting for the bus, and flicked rocks back into the landscaping in the sunshine.

Sunshine, giggles, a hug goodbye, and some small progress removing some rocks from the yard.

I will take it for now.

As my treatment plan expanded into weeks instead of days, months instead of weeks, it got harder to keep myself together.

It would have been so easy to put my head down, to give in, to just wallow into this process. It would have been less work, less energy, and just so easy to give into it.

Allow the chemotherapy, the drugs, and the exhaustion a place at the table.

I had my moments when I was weak, and sad, and I wanted all of this to just be done.

Would it go faster if I give in? If I caved to the madness of this entire experience?

It isn't in my nature—quitting. I am a fighter, I work through things, and experiencing thoughts like shutting down and crying make my heart physically hurt.

I like the word regrouping—it allowed me some grace in that in THIS moment I may feel like I am falling apart, but I can always regroup! Bring it back together. Pull it to me closer again.

And regroup.

I had begun to experience a new level of awareness in those few weeks. An awareness of things around me that I think I let go by me. An awareness that is familiar to me, but one that I have allowed to slide back into the reserves of my thought, drifting quietly until I needed it again.

That moment is now. It is time to become more aware of time. Of the world around me.

Of the little things.

One of the things that I appreciated learning during Frank's recovery from his traumatic brain injury was that the smallest things could either bring you joy, or bring you to your knees. I vividly remember the moment when I saw him quit, saw him give up, and how angry and sad it made me feel in that moment. I could not believe that the guy that I trusted to never quit on anything was giving up on getting better.

In that moment, I could see everything—his confusion and fear, his desire to just turn back time. I could smell the hospital room and the flowers that had been brought in, and I could feel the air blowing on me from the fan in the room.

The moment was locked into time for me, a snapshot of my life, and I knew that moment would be important to both of us.

I noticed everything right then.

I chose to shake him out of his moment, and yelled at a man who probably didn't deserve to be yelled at—but I was having a moment.

I asked him if he was a quitter, if he was leaving me after everything his team did to save his life—was he just going to give up? Quit?

It was a terrible display of drama from me, but in the end, it shook him enough that later that day he decided to walk for the first time since his car crash.

And from them on, he fought back to get better.

I want that to be me—I want to fight back. I want to get better.

I know that being overwhelmed is a natural part of going through cancer treatment, or dealing with a trauma, death or any number of life altering events. I understand that it is normal.

I just cannot figure out how to deal with such a cumbersome process—months of treatment and surgeries. I cannot wrap my head around so much.

But little things, small pieces of life, I seemed to be able to bring those in. Small moments, small events, that brought happiness, even for a second.

Those small events could turn the tide for me.

Sunlight. Giggles. Shooting goals.

Those small things can bring me back to life if I let them.

Breathing. Small levels of awareness.

Seems to me I found a tiny thread of hope within the events of those days.

Chapter Five

My nerves are showing

April 27

Today is the day before—the day before the last of this round of chemo drugs.

And I am nervous.

It is funny how I went into these in the past without too much worry. I think I am used to tackling things head on, and know that I am held in God's hands, so I don't worry about things much.

Today at work I had a lot to do so it was easy to move through the day.

But now, at home, there is time to think. And to worry.

I am not worried about the process, I am worried about how I will feel.

I just don't do sick well, and not feeling well makes me anxious. The combination of those two is not pleasant.

I have also been fighting an ongoing infection with my port, and came close to having surgery yesterday to have it removed. I am trying one more round of antibiotics and some strips to try and close the incision. Prayers that it works, as I truly want to keep my port for the next rounds of drugs, instead of having an IV every week for 12 weeks. Funny how something that I did not want is now something that I am trying desperately to keep.

I was humbled this week by two things, and I honor those moments in my heart as I head into tomorrow.

The first was the ongoing food support for the family. The meals, although hard to accept for me, are such a blessing. Knowing I can put that worry out of my head is more than anyone can know, so thank you to everyone that has offered and delivered food.

And to the angel that brought an entire shopping bag of berries to me today–you are my hero. There is nothing better than berries.

My second humbling moment came yesterday in the form of a bill. Yep, the first bill since this process started.

Knowing that I have had many tests, procedures, chemo treatments and drugs, can you guess what the current tally is that has hit our insurance?

Take a guess....

The number is staggering–$55,000. Yep. That is what it has "cost" so far to treat breast cancer. And I am nowhere near done.

Now, thankfully, I have health insurance. This is not what I pay, but the charged amount for everything done so far.

How can this be?

I am part of healthcare, and I get the costs, but how? What do you do if you can't afford this? I mean, who COULD afford this anyway?

Amazing number, isn't it?

It made me sit back and wonder how to make this better, how does healthcare truly function?

And how do people without it get what they need?

Bigger philosophical questions than I can answer tonight. I am just grateful I am in my home, with my family, trying to breathe and relax before another chemo session tomorrow. 4/4 for the big dog sessions.

The last of the hard ones.

Going to Ground

May 8

Going to Ground–This is the best description of where I have been for so many days post chemo. Where I went to figure out how to live through that time and how to come back out with myself intact.

Wow, chemo is hard. You hear it, you know it, but until you have truly experienced it, there is nothing like it that I have been through in my life. I will say that it is a process, and one that many people go through to get well. I understand that–but logic sometimes doesn't enter your mind when you are in the thick of things, and wondering when or if you will ever return to the you that you once were.

I look back on the last two months, and so many things have happened. Not just to me–I mean it isn't always about me. But life has moved on, even when I wasn't truly being a part of it. My kids are taller, two finished up college for the year and are either home or on to the next adventure, soccer season is in full swing, and the weather of sunshine has returned. School is coming to an end, and summer will be here shortly.

Life moves on, even if you don't.

So many people have asked me to describe how chemo feels. "You are good with words, how would you describe it?" Even I have been struggling to come up with how it makes me feel. Here is my best shot at trying to bring someone who hasn't been there into the world of chemo.

Have you ever seen Harry Potter movies? The later ones, with the dementors? Those scary, faceless creatures that fly by people and use their power to suck at people's faces, blurring them and taking away parts of their soul?

That is how chemo makes me feel—like I am blurred, not myself, and parts of me, and my aura, are being displaced by something that I have no control over.

It lasts for days, that feeling of being hit by a truck, poor awareness and engagement, and being out of control of you.

I hate that loss of myself, and towards the end of a week wondering if it will ever get better, or if there is really something wrong with me, it releases me back to myself, stripped of so much, but back.

I leave that time feeling stunned, and weakened by the experience of my being feeling stripped away. When I ask others, I am told that I look like myself, just like always, but I truly don't feel like me.

I come back slowly, with a new awareness of distrust and wariness, wondering if I will return to whole.

In the thick of things, the plans for eating well, praying, yoga and meditation fall to the side. It is a struggle for the survival of each day, finding a way to center back to yourself, knowing there may be things that can make it better, but struggling to make them happen.

I am grateful to be on this side of that chemo experience. I have completed that drug regimen, and am in limbo waiting for a scan and some information before starting the next 12 weeks of treatment.

For those of you praying for the healing of my port, thank you. It is a mess this weekend, and I have a feeling when they look at it tomorrow I may be spending the afternoon having it removed. My body has fought the port since day one, and I am not sure we can fight it much longer. There are no more antibiotics—just healing that needed to happen, but not sure that it we will get there. I will know more tomorrow.

Thanks to everyone that posted today that is walking in the Race for the Cure. I had no idea that people were walking for me, and the pictures just warm my heart.

Thanks also to my soccer family—the gift cards were a huge surprise and bring me such joy to know you are all thinking of me.

The journey continues.

Good news, good news, not so good news

May 12

I have written this post so many times this week–and as the week has moved forward, things have changed.

Here is the short version of a lot of things happening this week.

After recovering from that last round of AC chemo, I have finally felt like myself again. Energy is great and I don't feel like I am part of a Harry Potter movie anymore. Blessings all around on that! I had an ultrasound on Monday to measure any change in both the size of the lymph gland that was the trigger for all of this fun, and the tumor. The first batch of good news was that the lymph gland is essentially normal size, and the tumor has shrunk by half. Both great news to hear.

The second good thing was I had a revision of my port on Monday–the surgical line opened up, and it just would not heal, so they went back in and stitched things back up.

Tuesday I met with my oncologist again, and he was pleased with the reduction in size of the tumor and the lymph gland, and feels we should move on to the next phase of chemo. Thankfully, I got an extra week "break" and do not start again until next Thursday–another whole week of feeling like myself and being able to get things done was really exciting to hear.

Now the not so good news–Tuesday night my port started to get painful, and by today, I ended up back with Interventional Radiology for a check. The first things the PA said was "yeah, not okay." I feel like I spend more time worrying about my port than anything else. She consulted the surgeon, who offered to take it out today.

Since I had some things I wanted to get done this afternoon, I opted for tomorrow.

So the port comes out tomorrow with the goal to give my body a week without it. A new port will go in next week right before chemo starts.

Fun times with this chemo process–I'm just sayin.

I am grateful that I am on this side of the AC chemo–the Taxol is supposed to be easier, although 12 weeks seems like a long time.

But I will make it through.

Thanks for the cards that have come over the last week or two, they always make me smile. I am humbled by so many thinking and praying for me.

It is a break. Any break in the process was good, but an actual scheduled break was an amazing gift. It was time to think that life was almost normal (or whatever one thinks that life should look day-to-day). To being to find my footing again, to feel like I had some input into what will happen each day after I woke up—it is astounding to feel better, even if it is just for a short time.

I tried to practice the art of breathing. The art of noticing and paying attention.

The art of being grateful for each moment.

It sounds clique to me sometimes, "just be grateful for each moment." But you know what? When you truly balance yourself in a place where you can smile at the sunshine on your face, relish in the smell of flowers, and laugh out loud, life shifts into a new place.

A better place.

For the time being, I felt like my head was above water. I felt like I may be able to make it through the next 12 weeks with some ability to still function. After that, another surgery or two and I would be on the mend. A few more months, then with any luck cancer will be gone, I will have healed from surgery and recovered from chemo and radiation.

This would all, eventually, be behind me.

When I look back it was almost hard to believe that it had been four months. Four months on a crazy ride through Cancer Town. Months of doctors and appointments, months of a schedule even I wondered if I could manage, months of pain and feeling terrible.

It was hard to imagine still being in the middle of the storm, but I am there. I was still intact. I could still find "me" in all of the chaos.

The break is essential—I wonder if they scheduled it on purpose.

I know that not every giant change in life has a break. Sometimes when you are living through a storm in life it feels like it will never end. Divorce, death, dying, pain and suffering—these things are all around us, and many of us are living with them sitting on our hearts. A break would be a gift, but we don't often get a break—we are just expected to plow through whatever is happening, and still go on with the life that we lead.

Without a breather, how do we as humans, make it through these times, how do we not break?

Well, some of us do break. It gets to be too hard, and we go to our knees. Too many hits, too much pain, too much heartache can just take us down. Where do we go?

I go to my heart. Deep in my heart. To a place that remembers the sunshine. To the place that remembers the smell of the flowers, the warmth of the warm air.

The small tiny moments that allowed me to take another step forward—the gifts that I noticed before.

That is how we can move forward, a tiny step, a tiny moment at a time.

Being brought to your knees by despair. The longing of loss, the heartbreak of trauma can bring anyone to this place.

But we can bring ourselves out as well. Close your eyes. Feel the pain, acknowledge the hurt, the fear, the realness of this moment.

Breathe in the smells right now. This is also a moment to be remembered.

In this place of pain, invite the small joy in. Ask it to be present with you, to sit alongside you in the pain. The sunshine, the smell of flowers, the laughter of others. None of them have left you, they are all right here, waiting to be brought forward when needed most.

Even in the darkest times there are glimmers of sunlight. It is always there. Bring it with you.

I was banking some of this hope and joy that I had found. I was praying that I would not need them in the near future, that I could just enjoy knowing that I was trying to slow down and pay attention to life around me, to the small things that were making me smile and joyous, and to not worry about what may come.

I could not control everything, and I needed to stop trying. I planned to control how I reacted to the things that were to come, and I would remember that I had some sunshine hiding in my pocket if I ever needed to bring it out to brighten my day.

Chapter Six

Ready, Set...

May 24th

An eventful week and half for me on the cancer journey.

With the removal of the port, we thought things would settle down and heal up. Apparently my body had other ideas, and through the previous weekend, the now closed surgical site became increasingly uncomfortable. By Tuesday AM I was fairly certain that another surgery was in my future, and I came to work without eating breakfast. After a quick morning meeting, I headed down to oncology (have I mentioned how great it is to receive treatment where I work?!?!) and connected with both my chemo nurse and my oncology nurse. Both agreed the doctor needed to take a peek at it, and his expression when he saw how red and angry the site was wasn't a surprise.

So for the third time in 8 days, I headed back upstairs to the Outpatient Care Unit for surgery. They opened up the site, packed it, and left it open with a bandage on it.

And this is where we wait. I went back the next day for a change of dressing and packing, then visited the wound nurse a day later.

Here I was informed that this will not be closed up, and instead will be open and packed (by Frank and me) for the next 10-12 weeks.

Yep, gross open wound for weeks. Totally sucks.

I understand that my body rejected the port, but why it now is not healing up is discouraging. Not to mention gross.

Did I say gross?

Chemo was bumped out an additional week, and I am now two days out from starting chemo back up again. I was cleared today to go in and use an IV for the first couple of doses, since they are weekly, and then take a look at another option, either another port on the other side, or a PICC line.

Neither sounds like a great plan to me, but we will see how things progress, it has been great being away from chemo for the last few weeks—I would say I am at about 90% of my usual busy self, and it feels great to just be me (minus the red hair). Hoping to see some of that return with the lighter dose of chemo coming up.

Tumor is shrinking, I am healthy, summer is here and I feel good.

I will stick with that for now.

I'm just fine

May 27

I am fine—really.

I know many have been asking how I am doing after the first round of the new chemo, and truly I feel just fine today.

The process for this chemo is a little different than the last one, and of course, not having a port, that makes things slightly harder, but not terrible.

I always have to have labs drawn to check my levels on many thing before I get cleared for chemo. Doing so now requires a line being started, which is not nearly as easy as just popping an access into my port. Luckily, my chemo nurse is amazing and started the IV on the first try, and got my labs sent off.

Once they came back fine, I had to take another handful of drugs to prep for side effects–they are different with this chemo, and for the first two times, there is a risk of some pretty scary reactions. I was lucky to get all of these medications orally, instead of IV, as I hear that IV benadryl can be nasty. I then had to wait 30 minutes for everything to load into my system, and then start the new chemo medication.

Now this medication is an easier one, at a lighter dose, but there can be immediate and scary consequences.

Because of the risk of allergic reaction, the nurse sits with you for 20 minutes, and if you have any changes or weird symptoms, as a patient you have to say something quickly so they can shut it off and load you with benadryl and other medications to stop the reaction. So the minute she started the IV, and sat there and thought to myself "Is this a reaction? Does my chest hurt? Do I feel dizzy?"

This went on in my head for a few minutes until I decided that this was stupid, and maybe I should relax and just chat to take my mind off of things.

So I did. And nothing happened.

I made it to the end of the run, and went home with Frank. Other than being tired last night, which I was sure was due to the stress of the new regimen, and not to the meds, I was fine.

Today, I also feel fine, which is a huge relief and makes me feel that 12 weeks may not be too bad.

Now I know that this has the potential to accumulate and make me tired. But without all of the anti-nausea drugs every day, and how great I feel, I am hopeful that I can last many weeks without too much disruption to my life.

We made no plans for the weekend since I had no idea what we were getting in to, so I look forward to some time with the boys, and some gardening.

The port packing continues, now daily, and I can only hope that it continues to slowly heal during this time, and that there are no more complications.

I am grateful for this weekend, and hoping for the best in the near future. Thank you for all of the prayers and support, it truly helps.

Choices

June 3

There are so many choices to make every day. We choose what to have for breakfast, what to wear to work, what TV shows and games we allow our kids to watch, and what to make for dinner.

When a medical event enters your life, the choices become so different–life alters in a way so unexpected that when you look back, it is hard to imagine a time when the things that you got to worry about will ever be the same.

My daily choices still involve what to wear and what to eat for breakfast, but they are heavily colored with thoughts like "Will I be warm enough and should I wear fleece leggings today?" Do I have enough protein for my first meal?" Is this enough calories?" It is so interesting to have such a significant shift in thought process that one often doesn't notice it is happening until they get a reprieve for a little while.

My month off of chemo gave that to me, and I find myself working back into the more complicated organization of life living with chemo treatments that are now weekly. With my port wound slowly healing, I have that additional factor every day to think about as well.

Chemo session two went very well yesterday, and I was lucky enough to have Mariah, my wonderful daughter, with me so she could see firsthand how NOT scary it is. We had a pet visit, snacks and juice, and ate lunch together–not too bad a deal while having Taxol pumped into your system. My goal was to show her that the actual process of chemo isn't so bad, but I know I am lucky to be past the harder chemo drug, this one so far is easier, but has its own quirks to it that is for sure.

Each week I have to watch for fatigue, diarrhea and pain–the pain is neuropathy, which is painful tingling in my hands and feet, and if it starts, it could be permanent.

Fun eh?

Fatigue I understand, and have found that once I get home from work it is usually time to sit down for a while. The meals being delivered are still such a help–I hate giving up that control but it allows me to let go of the house control for just a little bit, and it gives me one less thing to think about. Life is already so complicated, I am grateful that small pieces can be moved away. Having a soccer schedule also managed by my friend Jenny has made all the difference in the world, and Jenny even texts me what is happening during the game so I can stay connected.

It allows me again to choose to rest, and heal.

The choices are endless, with the biggest choice of all is how to face cancer. I think it is easy to allow it to take over. Part of the process DOES take over with all of the appointments and procedures that you have to go through, it is highly disruptive to normal life and work, and I know how happy I am to have my treatment where I work; it certainly makes it easier. Not the case for many people that have to choose between working and treatment.

How can one do that?

On top of that, choosing what's best for you from a treatment perspective, and knowing what is the best choice–that is almost impossible to figure out.

I made the choice a long time ago to make the choices that would make sense to me, whether everyone agreed with me or not. Chemo, yes. Supplements, yes. Diet changes, yes. I also made the biggest choice that has the biggest impact, and that was to choose to stay positive. It is a choice, and even on the hardest days, of which there have been many, I work hard to choose good thoughts, knowing that this is a temporary part of life right now, and if I need to, focus on getting through one hour at a time.

The research supporting the choice of positivity is overwhelming with cancer recovery. It doesn't mean that I believe I will be magically cured at the end of this, but by choosing to think well, be well and continue to live life with a positive outlook, I give my body the strength to heal itself.

I could fill my mind with many things: I hate cancer. I hate chemo. I hate how tired I am. I hate the cost of these drugs. I hate the loss of control.

Instead I focus on the others: I am happy to have such great practitioners. I love my chemo nurse. I have friends and family that support and help me, even when I don't want the help. I can still work. I can still have time with my family.

It's all about choices, and what we tell ourselves. There are days that I want to quit, there are days that suck.

But I choose to look to the good, even if I have to purposely make that choice.

Genetics, wounds and eyelashes

June 9

I am sitting here at work, not working, hanging out in chemo. It is nice to be able to vacillate between getting things done on a chemo day, and to sit still and figure out what I need to get done. End of the school year, work, camp schedules and new job for Frank create such a whirlwind of activity that some days I can't even figure out where people should be at what time.

This week I got more information back regarding "how" I ended up with breast cancer. What I found out wasn't surprising, but was also not the best news in the world–I tested positive for the BRCA-2 gene mutation.

What is BRCA-2 you ask? Well, this is the gene mutation that is highly linked to breast cancer, and ovarian cancer if it is positive. With mine coming up positive, it solidified for me that plans to move forward in the fall with a double mastectomy, along with probable removal of my last ovary to reduce the risks of cancer re-occurrence.

Whatever I can do to make a positive impact to not go through cancer treatment again will be added to my docket.

In my head, I was already planning to make this happen, the big question now is the when, where and how much surgery there will be, but that won't be decided until after the chemo is completed.

More to come for sure.

The positive news for the week was that this stubborn port site is finally healing. For whatever reason, my body hated that port, and now it is on its way to healing, even while on the chemo. I was happy to hear that there is some hope that this could heal up while still on treatment.

Eyelashes. I know, weird topic, but when this all started I knew that you lose hair–all of it in some instances.

For me, I was okay with every bit of hair loss but the eyelashes. And lucky for me, I made it through the hard drugs without losing them. What a surprise then as my hair has slowly started to come back, that my eyelashes decided to make the leap! They are not all gone, but the 4 or 5 of them left look pathetic sitting there all alone. Thankfully mine have always been light without mascara, and it isn't glaringly apparent, but really?!? We couldn't just keep those??

Vanity isn't something I worry about–clearly sine I never wear my wig and go outside without a hat these days–but sometimes you just hope that something will escape the scourge and wrath of chemo.

Apparently not.

Oh well, they will grow back. Just like everything else (well, maybe not the boobs, pretty sure they don't grow back).

Happy Thursday (also known as chemo day!)

Another connected

June 12

It seems like every single week that I am connected with someone else that was just diagnosed with breast cancer.

I know that nothing has changed but my perspective, but there are so many of us, everywhere, that it is getting hard to ignore. Visits to my office, emails from friends, connections on Facebook and texts letting me know that they themselves, or a close friend/family member was just diagnosed.

Reading and research only compounds the worry and distress surrounding breast cancer, so how does one truly know the why and how this is happening to so many women? Why are there so many of us now—what is happening that so many have exposure to things that cause cancer, or have genetic mutations that make it happen?

It isn't okay—there are too many of us.

This has to change, and it needs to change soon.

I could always tell when I was starting to feel more like myself—I was thinking about the good things in life, I was focused on making myself better, healing, and stepping more towards being my old self than the current self. I found joy in the doing, and not as much in the being, but I think most of that was trying to just grasp onto life again.

I did not want to forget what I had learned about myself, about life, in those last few months. A part of me felt like I had been on a trip, away from my regular life, and while there, I learned a different way of living. A way of being part of the world, instead of living in my own world.

I noticed that as I started to feel better I began to lose perspective of what I wanted to do. I vowed to myself in some of those harder chemo days that I would always remember how it felt, and how I was able to grasp on to the simple joys, the moments that made me happy, and use those as lifelines when I felt like I couldn't go through another day of chemotherapy. I wanted to be able to continue with that process, but I was afraid that I might just move on with my life, jumping back into the day-to-day chaos that was my own personal whirlwind.

I wanted to remember the hard times. I wanted to honor the gifts that it brought to me, the awareness of who I could be when I take notice.

Sometimes it is not enough to want to make a change in how you want to be. Sometimes it takes something truly profound happening in your life to make a change.

It is like losing weight and eating better. It is easy to gear up for it, but when it gets down to the hard work every day, it is not so simple.

I knew I could not forget all I had learned—I needed to be more aware of life around me.

I was trying.

But part of me wanted to move on. To just forget the hardest of the days.

Chapter Seven

Slowing things down

June 25

I have made it through 5 rounds of chemo–7 more to go until I can get a break. I have been trying to keep up with life as much as normal, but this week I was given a mini lecture by my chemo nurse about priorities. She knows I am working full-time (she sees me in the hospital) and she asked how I have been feeling. Each day I am still feeling pretty good, but by the end of the day I am wiped out, which means I spend the evening down in bed.

We chatted about that, and she asked that I write down my priorities for the summer, and what things were important to me right now. She then asked me to write down the things that I am doing, and to see if those align.

Well, of course some of them don't, and what it does is put things in a bit of perspective for me.

I have limited energy–I know that.
I have limited time each day–I know that.
I want to try to do as much as I can each day–I know that.
I have to find a balance with work and family–I know that.
But, I am not doing that right now.

What I am doing is working a lot, and not much else. Typical for me. I get worried about not working, and the scary feeling that can bring, so I just keep working. I worry about time off, PTO, short term disability, all the usual stuff. I also know that I will be out for three months this fall, and that worries me too.

It is a control thing, and I am finding that my beginning of lack of control again as this chemo starts to slow me down is causing me to worry more and more.

Type-A control freaks like me do not like it when things outside of us take over–and I am going to have to start letting things be out of my control again.

And I just don't like it.

No one gets through chemo without any side effects, and I am no exception. I was just hoping it would be easy a little bit longer.

Time to start slowing things down a bit and giving myself permission to rest.

Such a hard thing to do....

The Real Deal

June 26

You can't deny having cancer–well, I guess you could but that is not a great way to ensure you live and heal.

I have never denied my diagnosis, but I have resisted the urge to give in to it. Trust me, it would be easy to give in–to be devastated and feel like life will end. In a way, life as you knew it does end, whether you choose to fight cancer or not.

You can't "unhear" metastatic breast cancer.

What I can do is fight against it, using the tools, diets and medications that I feel make the most sense for me.

They might not for others, but all of us in the cancer fight get to choose how we will engage in the battle.

My biggest ally is sunshine.

I am always cold–that is nothing new. I have always loved the heat, the sun and would rather be hot than cold.

I find the sun to be a healing source for me, and to be able to grab moments to sit in the sunshine is wonderful.

I may not get to go for a run, or lift weights or bike today, but I will give my body something that makes it happy.

Sunshine.

Feeling the fatigue

June 28

I am beginning to see the pattern in my life–get up in the morning and eat myself through the am (breakfast, breakfast number two, snack and then lunch). Work is productive, functional and usually engulfed in meetings.

I find that I start to become aware of time about 2:00 each day, and what I notice is that I am slowing down, not able to jump from project to project, and I start yawning.

Chemo is starting to force me to make some changes in my day.

By the time I leave work every day, I am tired. Tired enough that I look forward to getting home and resting–something that is not in my repertoire.

This type of chemo doesn't have a ton of hard side effects–I still have the chemo rash, but with my hair and eyelashes making a return, it is easy to think that things should be fairly normal each day.

I am finding that is not the case.

It is a slow depletion, but noticeable to someone that is used to running at 100%.

I know in my head that I need to slow down, but I am not sure where to cut things. My wonderful friend is handling most of the soccer driving, so the only other places to make change are work or home. Luckily, so far this summer home has held itself together, with the boys being a big help with keeping up on chores throughout the week. Although I haven't been able to do all of the gardening that I want, small things are getting done, and

I am happy with what has happened so far.

Work is going to have to give, and that is the scary part for me—work is where I feel needed and productive, and my balance in my soul is maintained by working. Finding a way to balance my soul and my fatigue is going to be interesting.

I am very fortunate to work with a team of people that want to help, even if I don't want them to—yesterday, one of my work partners stopped in my office and blessed me with a beautiful blanket that she purchased for me over the weekend. Knowing I am always cold, and how much I love blankets, she hit the perfect balance to tell me how much she cares. She also asked very nicely, in the perfect way, to let her help me.

I finally agreed.

This blanket is extra soft, and last night, as I fell asleep, I threaded my hands through the blanket, and fell asleep knowing that I have friends that will stay with me through this process.

I love my new blanket.

Time and Priorities

July 2

Time is the best gift–it allows you to do many things, yet it is something that most of us take for granted.

Time gives us space within the day to do the things that must be done, that we don't want to do, and the things that we choose to get done.

Time is often limited, either by our choices, our life or our inability to say no.

Yesterday, I was given the gift of time. I finally took a day off, and was headed to the lake to visit my parents.

My youngest Tommy and the dog were coming with me, and I was really looking forward to my own personal time.

My gift came in the form of a text, asking if Tommy wanted to go to the lake with his friend, instead of coming with me. He actually paused a moment, worrying that he promised to go with me, but clearly wanting to go where the Jet Ski was going to be.

Off he went–leaving me with a dog. And the gift of time.

I drove to the lake with the dog, and arrived alone. As I walked into the house I realized that I have never been here without the responsibility of others–and now, I have all the time in the world to visit, relax and just be.

What an amazing gift.

I know that I am tired, I know that I need to give myself time to rebuild and heal after each chemo session, but within our life, that is an extremely hard thing to make happen. Even when allowing others to help, which is difficult for me, it still is complicated. That is just how life is for us.

I think back to last year, and all of the things that were going on this week–we had just bought our new home, a house that would allow for Frank to stay with us in his own space, an entire level for my parents, and open space for everyone else. We moved in, and three days later everything came to a halt as my Dad was admitted to the ICU with severe COPD. He spent 5 days in the hospital, then came home to my house on Hospice.

The world was scary, and uncertain, and it was difficult to figure out how to make priorities–moving, emptying the old house, cleaning to sell, moving in, unpacking, all the while worrying about how my Dad was doing. Time was never enough, and when faced with severe health crisis of a parent, you think there is never enough time.

It is now one year later, and time is still a challenge, but for different reasons. Dad is still with us, and I get to spend this weekend with him in his favorite place–the lake house. There are no agendas, other than the jobs that he will have me do, and time stretches before us without the need to rush around.

Time is on our side–for the moment.

There will be no worries about cancer this weekend.

There will only be peace, time to relax, and sunshine.

And thanks to my friends and work partners that gave me this gift.

It's just too much sometimes

July 11

I planned to write an update days ago—I had another chemo session last Thursday, and there were some issues on that visit. I planned to put together a post, and then the world exploded.

I have had some busy days, and some sad days since then, and I was finally was able to sit down and let you all know where things are, and where things are going with this treatment.

Some of my labs are starting to fall outside of normal, but according to my team, I have quite a bit of wiggle room, a gift for being typically very healthy. I was cleared for chemo after my doctor visit, which focused on setting up surgeon visits and discussing lower back pain and new cysts. I have opted to let both of those go for now, since as the doctor and I discussed, the chances of the cyst or the pain being new pain inducing tumors is very small. My goal is to get through these last few rounds of chemo, and then to rest until surgery.

Chemo is becoming an interesting challenge—each week there is a little more pain, a little more difficulty getting an IV to stay, and a little more time needed to let the drugs run. This past run had to be extended to two hours, and have saline run with it as well to reduce the pain. I also had the IV in a tiny vein on the inside of my wrist, which was unpleasant. Thankfully I was able to finish the run, but with a definite review of how things are going for this coming weeks session. We will start the run with the drugs at half the rate with additional fluids, and hopefully things will go well. Not going well means that there will be quite the discussion about the next plan, I have 5 sessions left—and I don't want the PIC line. If I cannot tolerate the IV, I hope there are other options than the

PIC. I just can't imagine trying to deal with another port site, and the risk of infection and rejection.

I am getting tired–I hate admitting that, I hate acknowledging that. But I am tired.

Over the weekend, even with help, I exhausted myself, and ended up in bed at 3:00 on Sunday. I figured my regenerative powers would kick in and I would feel better today, but it didn't happen, and by 10:30 this morning, I knew that I needed to head home. I think between the fight against the cancer, the chemo, and my body trying to regulate itself, it just wore me out. Sleeping today gave me a bit more energy, but I can tell that the chemo is compounding and I am not going to bounce back as fast as I want to each week.

I don't like admitting defeat, and this feels a bit defeating. I know that many people take a lot of time off during chemo, but that is not my nature, and the possibility of that causes me more distress than being tired. It is coming to a crossroads, and I am not sure which one I will be following.

I do know that coming home, eating some lunch on the deck in the heat, and heading to bed for a nap was a really good plan.

Tomorrow is another day, we shall see what it brings.

One more down

July 14

Good labs.
One IV stick
Awesome visitor.
Made it through the chemo with minimal issues.
Only four sessions left.
Definition of a good day.
Now to rest.

Just a moment

July 19

I have just a moment to sit in the sun and remember how far I have come.

    Diagnosed with cancer to fighting for my life.
    Understanding priorities and willing to let things go.
    Taking care of others by first taking care of myself.
    Enjoying moments of the day rather than rushing through them.
    Giving to others as an incredible sense of joy and love.
    Cancer still lives in my world, but cancer is not ALL of my world.
    My days are filled with regular everyday things, and that is where my time is spent. Spending wisely in the places that matter and that I can make a difference—not in fret, worry or fear of the unknown.
    I will know soon enough.

Fun times

July 21

Woke up tired. Again.

Getting sick of the tired, especially when I have to temper my normal enthusiasm for life to ensure I can make it to the end of the day.

Labs were good for chemo today so I was lucky to know all was well, I'm just tired.

I got a mystery text offering a croissant delivery–how about that?!?! Wonderful seeing a friend that has a huge heart and brings me pastries to a chemo and work day.

In addition to my lovely croissants my beautiful friend-child came again this week and we got to spend a nice chunk of time taking before she heads out for vacation. I am still running into issues with getting an IV started but once in there is only mild pain since we thinned out the strength of the Taxol.

My friend Joy left after a bit and I caught up on some emails. I planned to head to a meeting but as the IV almost finished I started to have pressure in my chest. I let it go for a few minutes but then it became apparent it wasn't going away.

My chemo nurse looked at me when she came in and said "What??"

She is a smart cookie.

I told her about my new symptoms and thankfully she didn't use the BatPhone (also known as the rapid response team) but I did end up with an IV push of Benadryl (ouch) with some vitals and an EKG.

All was well

Sent home with instructions to rest.

Another night of pizza for the boys–thankfully they LOVE pizza so that rocks.

Now I sit in bed, watching 10 episodes of Chopped, with work and life things swirling through my head that I won't get done. That's the part I hate then most–the want is there but the energy is not.

Maybe I need an assistant.

Anyone want the job??

Listen to me talk all day, write it all down, and stop at Caribou.

Any takers?? Payment is in Caribou.

Hoping a good night sleeps pushes me through whatever this new symptom is and I can rise tomorrow better.

Goal is to NOT have to call ambulance tonight to take me in to the hospital–now that would be embarrassing.

Again.

There was an old commercial that used to play on TV—I remembered it showing in the winter, although I am sure that it played other times as well. It was the ABC Wide World of Sports broadcast introduction and in it they exalted the "thrill of victory, and the agony of defeat."

I was beginning to feel a bit like that promo on TV; I know I had it in me to win, but I was worried that I was going to be defeated.

I am an introvert—I spent most of my adult life not knowing that about myself, but when I figured it out, it gave me a lot to think about, and a lot to give myself a break on. I could not understand why I enjoyed public speaking, but not parties. Why did I enjoy working on a project with my peers, yet at lunch, I struggled to make conversation?

I gained my energy from time alone, it is what empowered me to work with people, treat patients, and generally be who I am in public. I loved my career and where I worked, which involved engaging with people all day long.

But it was not where I went to get my power, my energy, and my peace.

I found that in the garden, in the sunshine, with my children or just being alone. In those moments, my heart and soul are filled with energy, peaceful connections, which allowed me to do the other things that I wanted to pursue in my life.

What I am noticed was that my alone moments were needed for basic life things, like healing, breathing and sleep. No longer did my energy gathering moments rebuild what I had lost. Instead, those moments were used to slowly rebuild what chemo and fighting cancer had taken away. It was why I was always tired, and why work and conversation had become so trying.

If I had really stopped and took notice of what I was doing every day, I would have realized that if I had given myself more time, more quiet and rest, I would probably have felt better more of the time. I just didn't know how to stop being myself, the go getter, even when I needed it the most.

I didn't know how to NOT be me, and I think it was catching up with me. I needed to be less of who I normally was, and more of that person that I kept talking about that spends time in the quiet, in the peace, relishing in the moments of sunshine, instead of the one who kept running into the rain.

And not paying attention.

I kept telling myself that it would all be okay—that this was a temporary journey, a short time path that I would eventually be able to leave, and return to my previous journey.

But was that really true? Was life ever truly that same after facing cancer? After losing a spouse, a child? After trauma?

I didn't think that life was supposed to be the same after that. Life changes, and we are to change with it. I was just not sure how to move on, without letting go completely.

It felt a bit like a trust fall—and I was not sure if I trusted myself enough right then to let go of the past and just allow the future to unfold without taking some control.

Chapter Eight

Keep on going

July 25

Keep on going–that is my plan and how I want to finish up the last few rounds of chemo.

Yes, I promise, I am still resting. I get home at the end of the day and spend most of my time in bed. The boys have adapted and often come and watch TV up with me, or stop in and check in during the evening. Even with that, I notice changes and added behaviors into our world that are a true sign of stress for these kids.

I hate that we are living another scary life lesson, and although I don't think about it often, I wish things were not so hard all of the time.

I know I should be grateful that I am living with chemo, living with cancer, living my life even during a treatment protocol that is rigorous. There are others in my life fighting the same battle and not having positive results, and sometimes you wonder "Why me?"

Life is what you make of it, even in the hardest times. We all can choose how we react to the things that happen during our day–choice is often what makes the difference between a life-lived and a life loved.

I feel that love is a purpose, and a guiding force that can drive you to a wonderful place.

The journey continues...

One foot in front of the other

July 31

Every day now is one step closer to the end of the chemo rounds, but even knowing that, the steps are not necessarily easier or faster.

I find myself getting tired sooner in the day, earlier after chemo, and recovering less each week.

After the last round, I gave my chemo nurse a huge hug, and we looked at one another and said "only two more." It is amazing to think that I have been through 14 of 16 rounds of chemo through almost 6 months of treatment. Even with the hard, scary days, the really crappy times, the hair, eyelashes and eyebrows leaving, sickness, fatigue, weight gain, and loss of control over many parts of my life, I still feel like the time has moved very quickly.

I feel that the trick to this has been to continue to live my life every moment that I can–to continue the things that I love, just on a much smaller scale. Instead of gardening in my entire yard, I did a few planters, and bushes, and two important trees. Instead of going to the gym several times a week, I walk outside as much as I can, finish 20 squats, and relish in the sunshine each day.

I have found that it is important to notice the small things and take those instead of wishing for bigger and more.

Breathing in the smaller moments does shift the way that you see life around you. It is easier to relish in the lily and sunshine outside during lunch knowing that they are as important as a 5 mile run, a garden full of flowers, or a day full of busy.

I am strong, but I am tired.

I look forward to the next 18 days–I will take that first week off after chemo, then begin to move forward again.

PET scan, surgery planning, medication review–all things coming in the next month.

Blessings in Four

August 4

Today is a blessing–truly, all days we are here are a blessing.

Today I recognized the blessing in the number four, which surrounded me this week and settled in on this day, August 4th.

Today is my birthday–I feel that on your birthday you do things that make you happy, even when what is on your calendar might not be fun for the day.

I purposefully wanted to make this day memorable for me, so a few weeks ago I ordered 16 dozen cupcakes. On those cupcakes I asked that they be decorated with all the different colors of cancer ribbons–especially pink ones. Early this morning, I picked up all of those cupcakes and with my wonderful assistant (and super work partner) Jackie, delivered four dozen to oncology, four dozen to the breast center, four dozen to the infusion/chemo center and four dozen to the Rehab Institute. Each box had a note attached, asking everyone to celebrate every day, even the days that are filled with chemo or hardship.

I share this birthday with a great friend from Nepal and fellow law enforcement wives. There is no better day than your birthday to be on Facebook and watch all of the warm wishes and birthday celebrations flow throughout the day.

After the cupcake delivery fun I headed into my work day–four different meetings, checking in with staff, and a budget meeting scheduled for lunch. A meeting with another director ran a bit late so my boss stopped by my office to grab me for our meeting. I headed for her office, but was redirected toward my team's gym.

I knew something was up, and walked in to many members of the Rehab Institute cheering and smiling. I work with wonderful caring people, and today, pizza and pink balloons were just the ticket. Knowing the love and support that exist on that team makes it easy for me to be there, even on the days that I don't feel myself.

My four kids checked in all day long letting me know they were thinking of me, and after my "pizza budget" meeting, I headed to chemo. Chemo went great, and while I was there, I was given my own cupcake and a birthday song by the nurses, and then another rapping birthday song from two of my other teammates. All in all, chemo went quickly and I spent the rest of the day finishing up work and heading home to a dinner delivered by another great friend. The boys went off to play ping pong and I am now reflecting back on the information I received this week.

I got to meet my surgeon for the first time as we get down to the last two chemo sessions.

I always knew this was the next step, so it was a great way to start planning ahead to what was next. My doctor is a smart, fast talking energetic surgeon, and I appreciated her candor.

We talked about how I have been feeling and then we talked about the future. She started our planning with interesting news—she told me that most people with my diagnoses do not get to see her. I have seen many different diagnoses and descriptions in my chart, and she confirmed for me that I am considered to have Stage IV metastatic breast cancer.

With this diagnosis, the pattern of care and prognosis are not often aggressive, or geared to saving a life. The pattern of care is more stabilization. But my team, especially my oncologist, took the road of aggressive treatment, chemo, surgery and holistic programming. Although not surprised to hear this, I feel blessed that this is the road that was chosen for me, even when I know how hard it has been, and how hard things can be in the future.

This is not a good diagnosis—no one wants Stage IV cancer. But I feel happy, I have faith that each day has the potential for hope and fun, love and happiness, joy and passion.

I have not, and will not, let breast cancer take over who I am or where I am going.

Surgery is scheduled for September 15–I will spend a few days in the hospital and then a few weeks at home.

The surgery is not difficult for this experienced team, but it will be aggressive, and have risks that come with trying to remove as many risks of future cancer as possible. I will probably be recovering for four weeks, but my surgeon suggested that maybe six would be better to take the time and heal.

I will think about it :)

Next week is my last chemo session on Thursday–it will be the end of one part of the journey and the beginning of the next.

It was a wonderful birthday filled with laughter and joy, and as I told one of my teammates today, any time you get to have a conversation during the week that starts with "So what are your thoughts about nipples?" you know there can only be laughter ahead.

Reality and Realization

August 7

My reality varies depending on what part of the week I am in–Thursdays and Fridays are pretty good days, and my world shifts to slower speed and rest for the weekend and early week. Each week of chemo causes me to have more slow time and less normal "Lisa speed" time, but I know that this part of my journey is almost over.

In four more days, I will complete a chemo plan that was started way back in March. Although I cannot believe that it is over, I know that I have walked each day of this process with different memories, feelings, and left over scars.

Cancer has now been a part of my life for 6 months–and life has continued to move ahead as much as possible.

A few days ago I had a realization that made me really step back and evaluate my mental health. I was driving to work and listening to the radio. There was an advertisement for a walk/race for cancer, and I thought to myself "that is so nice." What I didn't do when I heard about the race was identify with the people that they were raising money for–I did not identify with having cancer.

I saw my doctor later that day, and I told him this story and expressed to him that I didn't think that I was in denial, but I truly felt that I have just chosen to take this treatment on as part of my daily life. He told me that he sees me as someone who has treated a very serious diagnosis as an addition to life, not as something that has taken over my life.

I was delighted to hear that by staying in the lane of my life, with the added sidecar of cancer, it has given me not only a way to continue to live well, but also the well-documented support of mental wellness and self-healing that occurs with a positive attitude and an internal dedication to finding peace and calm.

As I walked through some of my past journal posts, I can see the ebb and flow of the different treatments, days of fatigue, and ways that I worked to cope with this process.

I can also see that not digging into the true harder facts of a Stage IV vs Stage III diagnosis has allowed me to be free to focus on healing, regardless of what is happening in my body.

True to fact I feel pretty good. I am looking forward to chemo this week and coming to the end of this stage of the process. I am also looking forward to my PET scan to see how all of this hard work has impacted my body.

With that information, we will see how the next stage of this journey plays out.

I plan for the PET scan to be revealing in the sense that a three way hit to cancer works best–chemo, supplements and mental focus. Essentially body, heart and soul healing.

Thank you for the wonderful birthday wishes and prayers this week–chemo on my birthday turned out to be a wonderful day!

It's Over

August 14

It's over. Chemo is done.

It is hard for me to put a period at the end of that sentence because a piece of me wants to say "for now."

I think it is because I am 1% concerned about the PET scan tomorrow. So much of my heart and soul feels safe, mellow and not worried, but there is just a tiny part of me that knows that there can still be some concerns about cancer being elsewhere.

And truly, there is nothing that I can do about it.

If I have cancer in other places, or new breast cancer, then that's what I have.

It means a different treatment plan, and no surgery right away, but I know there will be a plan.

There is always a plan.

I may not know what the future holds, but I do know that it will come whether I feel I am ready for it or not.

PET scan here we come–early morning test, then off to work. Hoping not to have my Monday crash tomorrow but I know that it can happen, and if it does, then home I will go.

Short and sweet

August 15

News travels fast so I am just getting it out there.

My PET scan is clean—no active cancer anywhere!!!!!

On to surgery September 15th and taking my life BACK!!!

God Bless all of you for your prayers and support. This didn't happen by me alone—it takes a village and my village is the greatest.

Love to you all.

Kiss my ass cancer.

Breathing a little easier

August 16

Now that I have had some time to absorb things, I can start to process this time in my life. Being on the back end of a cancer diagnosis is odd–I think of the last six months of my life and it is hard to fathom everything that has happened.

Doctors appointments. Tests. So many lab draws. Surgery after surgery on my port. Pain. Feeling terrible. And chemo.

So much chemo.

But it's over–like everything in life, this has passed.

And I am at a bit of a loss on where my focus is now.

If I'm going to be honest, I am still recovering from the chemo last week. I am still tired, still dealing with the fun post-chemo stomach issues, and I still have my awesome chemo rash.

But I know, in another few days, my body will realize that there is no more chemo coming, and it will rejoice.

I have met some amazing people on this journey, some ahead of me, and some behind me on the same path. We are all warriors fighting the fight, and I am honored to be part of a group facing cancer head on.

Tomorrow starts the fight forward–and in a few weeks, a different battle when I head to the first of two planned surgeries to do everything possible to keep cancer from trying to come back.

It is what I need to do to be here for my family for a long time.

Looking forward to sleep tonight; tomorrow is another day, but for me, letting go of the fight mentality may take some time.

For now, I can breathe just a little easier.

I am not even sure how I got to this place.

This was a different place than I had been in for so many months—it was a stoppage, almost like it's over, but not over.

Part of this was definitely over.

To wrap my head around that fact that I had plowed through 6 months of chemotherapy, when at one point, before it started, I truly had no idea how I was going to make it.

What I found out, and I would now remember each day, was that no matter what is going on during any given moment, that moment always ends.

We can chose to either freak out or move through it.

I walked through each one, both the good and the bad. I remembered many of both, and when they were bad, I did not turn my back on them.

I let them enter into my awareness, greeted them, and then let them pass by.

Not denial, but coping in a way that allows the importance of even difficult scary part of our lives to have meaning. The pain and fear taught me lessons that I would not have learned if I had chosen to bury my head in a pillow and hide—instead, I took precious seconds with my sons, appreciation of sunlight and warmth, and found an ability to find joy and happiness everywhere.

I repeat, I was not in denial.

You can have an appreciation for tough times—especially when you work your way to the other side and can gain some perspective. The trick was to find a way to hardwire what you have learned into your life so you don't lose it. I bet it is really easy to move on with life and forget.

Forget appreciating the small things, the instances of short joy in tough times.

I felt that life would be better for everyone if we all spent a bit more time noticing the good around us instead of focusing on the negative.

I know it is easy to get wrapped up in bad stuff—I certainly had had my moments in those last few months, but I worked really hard to not go there.

How we react to everything in our lives is a choice; you can choose to be happy, you can choose to be mad, you can choose to flip off the guy that pulls in front of you in traffic, or you can let him be and be grateful you didn't hit his car.

We get to choose those reactions.

When you spend less time reacting negatively to things that happen around you, and more time appreciating the good, life changes, shifts into a new way of thinking. If you want to learn about positive thinking, feel free to Google it. Be prepared to find hundreds of articles, books and speakers promising ways for you to change how think and motivate yourself to be positive.

I don't feel that it takes another individual to make you aware of how different life can be. I do think that, unfortunately, it does take something traumatic or terrible for many of us to break away from our normal, typical life and reactions to said life. When something cataclysmic happens, it makes us sit up and take notice.

When these events happen, they can change us at a fundamental level, make us different somehow.

I am intrigued with this new part of me—I just wish I had not had to get cancer to make me more aware of the good. But I guess that was not up to me; how I choose to react to cancer and all the things that come with it?

Now that WAS up to me.

And I choose to be that different me that has emerged.

Chapter Nine

100% vs 50%

August 26

Does anyone ever feel 100%?

Does anyone feel like they are running at 50%?

Right now my head is running at 100%–I have been out of chemo for over two weeks, I feel good, and I want to grab life and sprint ahead while I have the chance. I face life like a fun challenge of events, and when life throws hardships at you, you need to figure out how to face them.

I feel like I face things with a positive attitude. I accept that life is difficult at times, and I have faith that whatever is brought into my life, I can deal with it.

My brain may be at 100%, but my body has not quite caught up with my brain. I wake up each day wanting to tackle everything on my list, and usually, my mid-day, my body is telling me that I need a break.

And my brain disagrees.

It is a daily struggle to remember I have limits–limit of energy, limit of food choices, limit of time in the day.

Making choices based on priorities, and the right priorities, is important.

In 20 days I will have surgery, and spend quite a few weeks recovering. I am comfortable with this decision, and truly, if I could, I would have surgery today. I am ready to move on to the next phase of this journey, but I will have to be patient.

Time for another tattoo, gaining energy and physical strength at the gym, and spending time with my family.

Blessing abound even in the face of many disruptions–like a broken air conditioner, furnace and water heater.

Who needs hot water anyway? It's still summer :)

Community

September 2

I think the word *community* means something different to different people. To me, community stands for those that are with you through life, whether they are blood or not. Community occurs when people around you work together toward common goals, creating harmony and fellowship together.

I have felt overwhelming community the last few months as I have recovered and those around me created a safety net for my family. Food, car rides, cleaning, and time were just some of the many gifts that we received from those around us. Our community involves very different groups of people, not linked by geography, but linked because of our family.

I don't often worry about the return of the favors we have been blessed with as I prefer to give rather than to receive. It took a long time for me to become comfortable with saying "yes, thank you, I would be happy to take what you are offering". And to know that we are held up in our lives a second time because of a major life event is a bit daunting.

I have chosen to be thankful, and I try to express that in many ways. Our community–family, friends, the kids school, my team at the hospital and law enforcement–are all a part of our lives, each one bringing us a different kind of blessing.

With the start of school just around the corner, I find again that the community reaches out, works together, and shares without asking.

In 12 days I will have surgery with the sole purpose being to reduce my risk of this or any cancer returning. If I could I would do it today, just to get the next phase of this process started. Instead I will be patient, getting life organized for my family, spending time with the kids, and knowing that my community is there with me.

I look forward to giving back to so many that have given to us, and to helping others say "yes" when offered help.

As my friend Jill taught me, saying yes allows others the blessing of giving to you; saying no robs them of their blessing.

I have learned to say yes, but I can't wait to help others say yes.

Time to Rest

September 10

Resting is not something I do well–even when I think I am resting, my head is still working hard to complete things.

I know that surgery may not be seen by most as rest time, but to me it will be a forced sit down of which I cannot avoid. Meds and pain, recovering and taking a break are all coming this week. The idea of taking it easy for 6 weeks is almost too hard to think of but I am sure my body will direct the pace.

I thought I would spend my few weeks between chemo and surgery getting things done and getting back to the gym. My head is working at 100% but by the end of the day my body is so very tired. On top of that I broke my toe, so any chance of spending time at the gym has gone out the window.

For me, that was the most disappointing event of the last few weeks.

I need time to rest. I know that, but it is hard to accept. I have stated that I did not want cancer to take over my life, and I fought hard to get where I am today.

Today I do not have cancer.

The goal is to keep cancer away–forever.

To do this, many of the significant life changes that I made at the beginning of this journey will be life long changes; Supplements, vegetables, minimal sugar and essential oils are all additional ways to fight cancer alongside medicine. My added goal once surgery recovery has occurred will be a ramping up of yoga, weight lifting, and more meditation.

It is amazing how much healing can be done within ourselves.

Sending healing to all of those on the same journey–so many have reached out to me as they start, end or continue their own fight against cancer.

Fight on everyone.

Time

September 11

Time goes quickly and slowly right now.

I want time to move forward so I can get on to the next phase of recovery. Yet I worry that there is not enough time to get everything done.

I sat on my bed today, making lists and schedules, trying to put everything together before Thursday.

Surgery day.

When I lean back, take a break, look at the sunshine filtering in, I know that I can't do everything.

No one can.

I know that in my head all will be well, but the tiny worry has started. I try to ignore it, but it has started.

I just want to get to the healing part.

I'm tired of feeling tired and sore. I want to just do what I want to do with my life, instead of tempering it to the "cancer" reality of energy.

I know it will come. I know it is another short price to pay to get my life back.

I'm just a bit over it right now.

Positivity can do wonders for you heart and your soul.

It can make you feel like you are 10 feet tall, can carry the world; positivity makes you wonder how you ever thought there was a bad day, or a hurtful remark.

It can shape how you feel, how you react, and how your mind works.

Positivity can change a lot.

It can also drive you mad.

Now this time I was referring to those around us that scream "I AM HAPPY" all the time, and they want the rest of us to be happy too.

As I read through my most recent sharing, I felt that I was coming across as the worlds' biggest happy cheerleader, rah rahing until curing myself of cancer. Eeeks, that really was not how I intended to become, but it appeared that I was there.

I continued to believe that there is truth to the saying "There is power in positive thinking." We know that plants, when either talked to nicely or yelled at, grow well or start to wilt depending on what they are exposed to. Just like that plant, when our brain is flooded with endorphin supporting positive comments that make us happy, we feel better. Does that mean that everything is perfect in our world? Certainly not. But it can make a tough time easier.

Compare this to a funeral—I am fairly certain that it is tough to find too much joy at a funeral (unless you really do spend your life being bitter and angry). Funeral, by nature, are often sad affairs.

Unless you are part of our family. Yes, there are tears. Yes we will miss the person that is no longer with us.

But remembering one lost can also bring laughter, wonderful stories, and bring people together for a common love for that individual.

Even a funeral can be a time of joyful seconds.

Each second counts.

Like pennies, they may not seem like much at the time, but when you look back at all of them together, they certainly do make us richer.

Chapter Ten

Pain and Recovery

September 18

Okay, yes, this hurts.

It is not as if I did not expect pain, but since I have not had much pain the last seven months it is hard to work through it.

With this process, there are two types of pain–physical and mental. The mental pain I have been purposeful in dealing with since the very beginning; mental focus, prayer, meditation and breathing work wonders for mental struggles. I am a firm believer in the power of the mind in making changes not only in the mental state but in the physical realm as well. I believe in connections to others, and using those connections for good.

I have been blessed with an amazing group of people that surround me and help strengthen my resolve.

Physical pain is different–physical pain can truly knock you flat, take your breath away, and wear down your resolve. Although the pain is not so bad I can't function, it certainly is not pleasant. But I am not sure it compares to another part of the mental pain that comes with this phase of breast cancer treatment.

The reality of significant changes in body appearance.

Those pictures you see when you Google breast cancer surgery are real—and although I did research, I watched the surgery, I knew what it would look like, I did not know what it would FEEL like.

Like I am not me.

Now, I have stated from day one that I did not need reconstruction, did not care about appearance for appearance sake. Flat chest, no chest or new chest, I was not worried about that part of this process. I want to focus on the health, not the appearance.

But the in-your-face reality of breast removal is much harder than the preparing for surgery reality. It is hard to know that your body has been cut apart, dissected, and now heals as it prepares for more surgery to repair and put it back together.

I was not ready for that part of this—feeling like Frankenstein.

If I am honest with myself, I think I would say that the physical pain mirrors the mental pain that so many women feel living through this reality—the pain of knowing that you will never be the same after this diagnosis, and parts of your body will forever be scarred while trying to fight for your life.

I wait—the healing will come, slowly, but it will come. The pain will receded, the drains will be removed, and I will prepare for ongoing surgeries and adjustments that will hopefully lead me to a clean bill of health.

Waiting for pathology reports is hard.

Waiting for the pain to recede is hard.

Waiting for more surgery is hard.

The new perspective is difficult, but it is real. I know it will get better, but I am impatient. Resting is not easy for me, but I am trying.

Thank you for the cards, and kind words, for checking in and for telling me it will be okay. The warriors ahead of me are amazing women, and I feel lucky to have their guidance as I keep moving forward.

Bored is better than Pain

September 21

Being bored is better than being in pain–but not by much.

I got busted today while purging my work email–there is not much else to do in a world where you have no endurance, have limited ability to move around, and are supposed to be resting.

Resting is not something I do well.

I am trying though, just as my mothers have told me to do.

Many of you know that I grew up in one of those neighborhoods with yards connected together with no fences, parents that sat on the deck before dinner for a drink, and lots of "family" holiday get-togethers. From this I was blessed with not one, not two, but a total of three mothers. And lucky for me, two of them spent their careers as nurses, one of them an oncology nurse.

What this means for me is a visit immediately after surgery to ensure that I am being taken care of properly, and a daily boob inspection to make sure drains are working, incisions are healing, and I am not exerting myself too much.

You can't find this kind of love anywhere people–no other love like strong, smart women in your face.

As I feel better I get antsier. Lucky for me there will be additional procedures that will bring pain back to my universe, and slow me down again. Funny how that happens...

Looking for some things to do to make my brain calm down–I will finish my painting and then start to look for something else fun. And quiet. Gah, can't I just go to dead-lifting again?

No? Really?

Back to the television...

Perspective 2.0

September 26

Perspective is everything, whether you are on the good side or the bad side of things, it is important to be able to see both sides of almost everything.

If we cannot do that, we are blind to many truths in our world.

My perspective the last few days has been bleak–this is the opposite of how I usually see the world, and different than I want others to see me. However, when the body and the mind are at odds with one another, it creates a dis-harmony that can lead to negative thinking and distress, even to those living with peaceful hearts.

Fatigue and pain are both bridges to the darker side of the mind. Even if life isn't easy, these two components of our world can edge you forward to a place that you don't want to go; a path that leads to harder times instead of light.

I recently read an article about individuals with exceptionally high IQ's and how their world had certain components that truly made them happy and that these were often not in align with what the rest of the world saw. Socialization may have been a negative for them, but thinking creative thoughts, organizing complex tasks or create beauty brought them joy and peace. Many that I know living with hard, complicated lives often seem happy and engaged in their days, even when living in what may appear to be chaos and hardship–for them, those are not the things that bring them down. Being unable to express, think, create or work are the things that destroy that balance of who they are, the things that bring them joy.

Their perspective is what allows them to have delight and joy in the days where others only see hardness.

Idleness is my hardship–lack of purpose towards others, giving of myself or inability to make good are what drive my life.

What may seem like a time of rest and relaxation is actually physically painful and hurtful–and may be doing more harm than good. There has to be a balance between rest and doing, breathing and creating, sleep and helping.

My balance is grossly disrupted, and it is causing more bad than good. Finding that balance again is paramount to me being able to remain healthy, and I am not finding it yet.

I miss writing, working, being part of a team, and watching others flourish and grow. Although there is much good in the day, it is hard for me to see the good while floundering with my brain fighting against that lack of getting things done.

Here is the list of the good: pathology came back with only 2/10 lymph nodes with cancer in them which was great news, tumor is gone with clean margins, my surgical sites are healing very well, and so far no signs of lymphedema or problems with my left arm. I have weekly visits to the doctors to make sure things continue to move forward, including another surgery next week to remove my last remnants of being a girl (just kidding really, who needs an ovary anyway).

I know this sounds negative and bitter, and truly I do not live in either of those places. I miss work, and sitting is hard for me. I should be grateful that I am healthy, cancer free, heading in the right direction to getting back to work, the gym, and getting to meet new people soon, but right now, in this moment, I am not at my best.

I am blessed, lucky and healthy, but sometimes the soul still isn't full.

It is hard to do for others when your body won't allow you to do for yourself.

Frustrating...

Water journal

October 2

Water is the best way to describe where I am right now on lots of levels.

First and foremost, I'm in the tub so I can "prep" for surgery tomorrow. There is now a special shower you have to do to reduce the risk of infection.

Fine with me–I like the water.

Water has another explanation for me in the way that I feel, which is a bit like drowning. I know that seems ridiculous–I'm not working, I have all the time in the world to do things, yet these are the times for me that are the hardest.

Some people thrive in organized, regimented routine of life. Work. Pay bills. Kids to sports. Dinner. TV. Repeat.

I do not. I relish in the chaos of multi-tasking, over-doing, project overload life that is mine.

Usually.

When it isn't, like right now, I flounder like a fish OUT of water. I feel that God gave me the gift of being a doer and a giver, and when those gifts are not used, it's almost sinful to my soul.

Now, I am in no way able to do all of that right now, and I give myself sometimes hourly affirmation that it's ok to slow down right now.

But tell that to my brain.

Someday someone will study people with ADD and realize that when channeled correctly, the world is a place of infinite possibilities. I love that. It makes me happy.

Today I was able to revisit our TBI website and do some updates about why we vanished for the last 8 months.

That felt good. It felt productive.

It made me feel less lost.

Breast cancer is all consuming–doesn't matter where you are in the journey, it just takes over.

I am plotting my revenge on this lost year–more presentations next year, back to the gym and hopefully joining a team of BC survivors, and telling cancer to kiss my ass.

My life has meaning and purpose.

We all have that purpose.

Sometimes we just get lost in the journey.

Lost was a good way to describe how I felt. It was almost painful for me to be idle, and although my self-talk was full of affirmations about how I was letting my body heal, apparently my head didn't buy it.

My head wanted to go and do anything that did not involve lying in a bed and letting others run the world around me.

There were the times when I realized that it was not so easy to do your best, find good things in each tough thing, to be the person that I always said that we can always be.

Definitely a "put your money where your mouth is" time in my life.

I still believed that it could be done, and I was committed to finding more excellence in my days, and I felt that anyone can do that, but sometimes I wanted to tell my own brain to shut up. It is like dieting, you know you shouldn't eat cake, but screw it, sometimes you just want cake.

A part of me wanted to bitch and moan about this current surrender to idleness, and the other part of me wanted to shake my head and say "get real."

So which side was winning out? Similar to chemo and my other resting moments, I was fighting with myself.

The good thing was that this is real—the fight to try to be better, to do better or different in our lives—is really hard.

Stopping a bad habit, learning a new one; both take the same amount of commitment. I appreciated the realness of things, and I could, in my head, put it in perspective of how when we want to change, it can be a real struggle. It doesn't matter how disciplined we are, focusing on ourselves and living the best that we can is really hard.

I want people to believe that these types of events in our lives can be useful—cathartic even—it takes a commitment to honor what is happening, and to then allow yourself to feel. As I continued to try to do that with my own experiences, I wanted others to find this level of connection to how we can be as people so much sooner than I did. It took a brain injury for my spouse, and breast cancer for me to finally be able to find pause in my life.

The pauses allow the moments to happen—the ones that we love, and remember, and allow us to realize we can do so much with our time, so much more.

It was easy to sit here, resting, and think about all of the things that I wanted to do with my life.

I wanted to continue to connect with people in a way that was positive.

I wanted to write more.

I wanted to spend evenings outside, in the garden.

I wanted to go to the gym and eat well all of the time.

I looked at that list and I thought "all really great things, Lisa. But how will you do that? How will you make life more about these things than the day to day? How will you commit to this?"

I am not sure, but when you are stuck in bed, it is really easy to think about what I WANT to do.

I was living in the thick of those choices, and not choosing as wisely as I would have liked to.

Lucky for me, my body shut me down before I could do too much harm, but I was watching, almost from the sidelines of a sporting event. I watched my inner conflict with amusement, as I thought about being a daughter that used to fight against my parents, and a parent myself watching my children doing the same things that I used to do.

You get both sides—sometimes choosing the logical better one can be trying.

I could only make plans at this point, and start at a place that both my body and my mind could cooperate together. Finding that happy middle ground was going to be tough, but the second half of this journey should be easier than the first half.

And then I could move on.

Chapter Eleven

Two weeks ago

October 18

Two weeks ago I had a plan–of course this was MY plan but I didn't feel it was unruly or excessive, but felt like continuing to move forward with each step of my breast cancer journey is important.

I wasn't afraid, I was organized.

I wasn't pushy, I was planned.

My breast surgery went well–boobs off, expanders in. Obviously it's painful but you adjust to those type of changes in knowing that each day is a tiny step forward in the process.

After some recovery time, which in real time was about two weeks ago, I went in for one of the last procedures that needed to be taken care of–having my ovaries removed.

With my breast cancer technically gone, doing the things that would keep it at bay were now very important and this would be a simple part of that process.

Or so we thought.

With any surgery there is risk–risk of infection, risks of difficulty risk of complications. There are usually many.

But routine operations for a much larger problem don't typically worry me, especially when I am fighting a battle and to me this was a skirmish behind the high school.

But in fact it was not.

A small simple procedure turned into life threatening major surgeries, most of which I was blissfully unaware, getting to ride it out on a ventilator.

But many of you were not unaware–in fact the absence of information and lack of updates caused many of you a lot of fear and pain and for that I am so sorry. I consider my verbal outspokenness something as a helpful tool but it clearly left a hole of the unknown when not in use.

It is surreal to be talking about something that I have no memory of, which gives me a new appreciation for how hard it is for humans like my husband, who have a brain injury, to know that they don't remember a part of their lives. It is scary for sure.

Here is what I know based on what I have been told.

The small surgery seemed to go fine. I went home, had some pain and moved on. But a few days into recovery pain became a huge problem and I returned to the hospital—I remember arriving and telling my husband to go home, knowing that I would probably get some pain meds, a long wait, and then get to head home.

I remember texting my mom, and I remember telling the doctor that I was sure I was being a big baby. I remember telling my mom I needed a CT scan.

And then I remember nothing.

What I have been told is that I continued to text family and friends. And then the shit hit the fan. A perforated bowel had occurred days before, and I was rapidly deteriorating. My mom was told to hurry to the hospital to assist with making decisions on how far to push things. Surgeries to fix the leak, to resection my bowel, more surgery, a ventilator, and some very scary times for my family.

Luckily it took several days to come out of my drugged up state to understand the scariness of the situation. A significant bowel bleed that needed multiple types of surgeons and months of recovery.

I couldn't believe it—so much for my plan, eh?

But this is how life works; we make a plan, move to execute and adapt along the way. For me, this process and change will be my huge adaptation to recovery, and hardest in the fact that I will personally need so much help for myself for the simplest of things.

But as always, I have a choice. I can be pissed this happened and spend my very limited energy resources in the Book of Angry and Irritated, or I can look forward at the now baby steps that recovery will take to get through this.

I choose the harder path—I choose the baby step, slow down, not always on my terms mode of recovery.

Because the Book of Angry and Irritated is destructive, and I enjoy building things up, not taking them down.

Energy will be put to moving forward and healing, and nowhere else. If you are currently reading the book of angry in my honor, know I love you for your support and passion. But let's go on a walk together in healing, in the sunshine when we can, and we can find a different book to read if we need too.

Right now I would like to get home, take some of those baby steps, and think about my cookie dough list that soon has to be started.

Healing with all of you is my own private peace and joy party, and I am lucky to spend it with all of you.

Another day here

October 22

Well we shot to get home yesterday and with Frank super sick with a head cold and trying to get everything moved in the house we let it go, and planned for a 0900 return home this morning.

Best laid plans...

Pain started to increase about 2000 last night and narcotics and exhaustion finally let me cave in about 0100.

Pain plan needs a good tweaking, which has already happened this am, and I will need to hang around to see if it works. Truly I am grateful I did not go home–I would have been right back in here last night.

I'm sad because I just want to be home, but even as I write this note, this level of pain doesn't work. I'm supposed to move, rest and recover–not freeze in place and hold my breath hoping the pain will get better.

So maybe today. Maybe not.

I have always said that pain is the great equalizer—it breaks you down like nothing else can. Right now I appreciate great medical care and pain relief. I am not sure how to even wrap my head around all of this, I just know that the small steps now will be tiny, and I am not sure I can think that far ahead.

The Fear of Silence

October 29

Silence is not always a reason to worry, although as a mom I can tell you when I am not getting a response from one of my kids I certainly start to feel that nagging feeling in the pit of my stomach.

I am also aware that silence from me, not a common thing, can also make people worry, and I am sorry for that.

After 15 days in the hospital, I returned home last Sunday to the reality of a home wound vac, nursing care, and pain management. I knew that it was going to be challenging, a new level of medical need and complication, but I am not sure that anything prepares you for the reality of where I have been in the last 5 days.

Difficulties started with the wound vac losing the seal the first day. Not unheard of but another thing to deal with. Most people are not familiar with a wound vac, it is a way to heal large open wounds faster, but it requires changing every other day by a nurse. When I mean changing, I am referring to dismantling of the packing and resealing the entire thing with suction.

Unpleasant.

Juggling wound treatment, med management, pain control, bowel function, eating to heal... it seems to never end and takes up my entire day–which is exhausting.

There are moments that I seriously wonder if I can do this–and I remember having the exact same thought as I started to go into labor with my youngest child.

It isn't a matter whether or not you can do this–it is how are you going to do it.

No one plans for complications, and as I think back as to how I expected this part of my breast cancer journey to go, where I am never even crossed my mind. Never did I expect complications so severe that I would have months of recovery added to my life, and a level of ongoing pain that would begin to drain the light from my soul.

Seem a little extreme? Maybe, but I am reminded this week of the impact of pain on a body, heart and mind.

Pain has the ability to pick apart our very being, impacting every small crevice of who we are, and after a while, you begin to notice how depleted you feel.

The lack of sunshine, the inability to move around, ongoing pain—I have yet to find a way to balance myself in this reality.

I am very honored by the thoughtful, kind gifts that I have received this week. Bright blankets, bath salts, lotions, charms, bracelets—the list goes on and on. Each one sent to me full of kindness and love, and I cannot tell you how wonderful each one makes me feel. Those cards, emails and texts are what are holding me together.

Today has finally given me a slight glimmer of being able to breathe slightly better, slightly easier, and I am hoping that it is the beginning of feeling better. I am tired of hurting, but more tired of the incredible disconnection from life and living. I am just not in a place yet where I can do enough to feel good about the day, but today there was a small window into the future that might lead to a reconnection.

Thank you again for the food, the support for my family, and the constant checking in—it truly does give me hope.

I am still here, resting, breathing slowly, trying to reconnect myself to the world.

A new discovery.

I could only think of this impossible situation as a new discovery in my life of patience and meditation.

And huge amounts of painkillers and television.

Truly, I almost didn't have the capacity to see more than a few hours ahead in this life.

"Is this how dying feels? A disconnect so hard from the future that you feel that you can only see a few feet in front of you instead of years?"

I knew that this would get better. I believed that I would heal, that all of those months of chemo were not for nothing.

I just struggled with the reality of pain.

I was also beginning to worry about how I could get better when all I could do was sit here, walk a bit to the bathroom, and maybe to the kitchen, and then return to bed.

How long would I be stuck in bed? How long would I be hunched over like an old troll? I felt like even standing up straight was too much right then.

I didn't know how to not be me, but this person, this sick person, seemed to be taking over my life, and I wanted the real me to come back.

I could feel the worry of losing myself completely starting to creep back into my heart—I was worried about losing who I was when my cancer treatments started. Now I was worrying that as things seem to have spun out of control, that I might not be able to find my way back.

I found a new respect for individuals that have met major life disasters and lived. And moved on into the next part of their lives full of renewed focus. Goals. Changes that they used for good.

I wanted goals. I wanted a renewed focus.

I wanted to do good.

Finding that my ability to think ahead had been reduced to planning what to eat for a snack or when my next nap would be had been disheartening. Pulling myself back up seemed a herculean task at that moment—at times my mind started to work on what could be, where life could go if I could just grasp a thread of the future.

And then it was gone.

Rallying would be my biggest achievement. Starting to find the tiny specks of a future life in the sunny moments of each day would have to be a start. It was like finding a needle in a haystack; you know that somewhere in the pile there is the one thing that you want to try to find, it just feels like more that you could possibly tackle.

But each piece of hay that is removed is one step closer to the last piece of hay.

Each moment that ticked past was one step closer to healing. Closer to renewed strength. A step forward is a step forward—do not disregard the tiny steps.

They are like those pennies again, one is not much but a 100 of them are a dollar. It all adds up.

In light of my ability to measure things in tiny pieces, I decided to make sure to pay attention to each of these small measures of progress. It did become amusing when I realize that I was looking at myself in the mirror and giving myself credit for washing my face AND brushing my teeth.

It was all about the little things.

If you had to find three small things to appreciate from today could you do it?

It still amazed me how much time we let slip by in life without takin a notice of it.

Chapter Twelve

Limits vs Strength

November 10

I started this post yesterday, and just could not finish it. I have met my limit, in more ways than one. It doesn't mean I have given up, but eventually everyone hits the end of their ability to keep their head up high and spout positive words.

I am apparently at my limit.

Another hospitalization, another week of feeling sick and tired, and I am over feeling sick and tired. This is typically where I stand up, fight back and push forward, but I am finding it difficult to dig deep and find the energy to do that. I am tired–tired of the limits, tired of the pain, tired of feeling crummy, tired of not being part of life.

I think the hardest part of this process is that my life is service focused, and I am now on the other side of that coin–instead of serving, I am receiving. I like working, I like helping others, I like being part of a process to make things better on different levels, and being pulled away from that life mission, and into a life of taking instead of giving can cause true mental anguish. At times it is physically painful for me to say yes, thank you for your help, the ride, the food, the gifts. It hurts me to take, instead of give.

I think that this the hardest part for me, knowing that I am sidelined for so long, by something that was completely unexpected. I am frustrated by the time it is taking to heal, and the need to do, give, work and help is so strong that when I am unable to do those things, it depletes my soul.

I am grateful for those that continue to be there every day to take me to appointments, support my kids, bring meals and just be there for our entire family. We would never have been able to maintain any sense of normalcy without all of you.

I know that at the end of this very long process that I will be able to return to my normal level of chaos, filled with work, kids stuff, engagement with others and giving. I know that there is a light at the end of this very long tunnel–but lately, it has been very difficult for me to see. There is a difference between our cognitive ability to know that things will be okay, and what is happening in our hearts, where we feel the sadness, pain and frustration of a situation.

I KNOW it will be okay, but my heart just hurts.

Marching on

November 15

I have successfully stayed out of the hospital for a week–I think that makes me think things are slowly moving forward, even if it feels like not much is changing.

I know that time is needed, I know that I must be patient, I know that I will heal.

But what I know and how I feel are not always on the same page.

I am grateful that the pain has slowly gotten better, and that I can continue to reduce the pain medication, which is certainly not helping my current stomach unhappiness. I am living with a chronic low grade nausea, which for me, is almost worse than pain. I hate being nauseous, and when nothing makes it better, it sucks. Eating, not eating, doesn't matter, it seems to always be with me. I am disappointed since I made it through months of chemo without any major stomach issues, and now here I am with bowel issues because of the complication and surgeries.

Very irritating.

I am dutifully doing my exercises to reduce the impact of the mastectomy (I am trying to make my therapists proud) and slowly moving around more in the house. Dealing with surgery recovering on several different parts of my body enhances the difficulty of things, and I am not even sure which is harder at the moment the ongoing expansion or the large wound recovery.

Neither of these are much fun.

I had another meeting with my oncologist last week and he did recommend radiation, hormone suppression and a possible clinical trial medication, all to help reduce the chance that this nasty cancer will come back.

Right now I am saying no—no to the clinical trial and no to radiation. Hormone suppression, maybe.

I just can't. I am maxed out and when talking with my mom, she had a great point. Her opinion was that there is only so much a person can take, and sometimes it gets to be too much.

I agree, it's just too much.

I am struggling going to my appointments and getting through wound care three times a week. I just don't want anyone touching me—it is more than I can bear some days.

I know that some of this is absolutely necessary—wound care is a non-negotiable. The rest of these appointments? Some days it's fine, and other days it's not.

I know I need to keep marching on, that there is light at the end of this part of the tunnel. It is just hard to know there are so many days left of recovery, when I just want to be back doing what I do with my days.

Marching on, marching on...

Pain-The Ultimate Equalizer

November 29

I have been quiet–more quiet than usual. Although still roaming around on Facebook, I have not had the energy to write a blog. There have been a few stops into the Emergency Department, and lots of calls into the clinic, but today finally wrapped up a lot of worry for many of us–proving again that prayers and support can truly lift you up.

The biggest issue has been the pain–I have had multiple moments of pain that truly took my breath away, which is scary.

I have not allowed myself to be afraid during this process–for a long time, I did not acknowledge that there was ever anything to worry about. As we all know, this is not true, and parts of this process there has been some very serious and worrisome times.

My goal is to only allow real worries to be part of my thought process, and not to worry about every little thing.

I am allowed to worry about pain.

Pain has been getting worse–so much worse that I ended up in the Emergency Department Thanksgiving night. I missed the turkey and the dressing, but the pain went away. When the pain returned, it was worse than before, and definitely time to see the doctor.

But of course it was a holiday weekend.

So Tommy and I rode up north to the lake with Grandma and Grandpa and got to watch the snow and sit by the fireplace. Tommy worked hard moving wood and making cookie dough, and I relaxed by the fire and took multiple naps.

Returning home meant preparing to go see the doctor, and by that time, I was scared about what they would find. I could not even touch parts of my abdomen where the wound was, and in my head, the more pain there is the worse the wound is. To be honest, a lot of very scary thoughts went through my head.

My visit Monday with the Physician Assistant was filled with tests and a debate on whether or not to be admitted to the hospital.

My pain was clearly not under control, and it needed to be. Pain slows down healing, and that is the opposite of what we want.

Ultimately I opted to head home with new pain meds, and went to bed. I set four alarms to ensure that I woke up to take my pain meds so the pain did not get ahead of me. What I was really waiting for was the appointment today, which I was truly worried would lead to more surgery.

The surgeon I met with today I had not met before–he was incredibly calm and engaging, and I was immediately set at ease. Of course he needed to see the wound, and the painful process of taking the dressings off had to happen. Once that was done, he spent quite a bit of time talking me through the different things he was seeing, spots that I explained were hurting a lot, and how things looked to him.

In the end, he was quite pleased with the process of how things were healing, and what he wanted to do next.

I felt appreciated, listened to, and like a very special patient. He walked me through each new step, and how quickly he felt things would move forward with this new plan. Pain, which is still quite a factor, will continue, but not in a bad way. This type of pain means nerve endings are coming back, and I am feeling that growth.

Some shifts with pain meds, and some new taping process, and things should get back on track quickly.

My fear is reduced, pain is present, but I am relieved.

The prayers and support have always given me peace, and today was no different than any other day. Thank you for giving me the strength to get through the last few weeks–these were some of the hardest times ever, and your support is why I made it through.

Blessings to you.

Good day Bad day

December 10

Such a toss up–I never know what I will get. I know so many have many more problems than I do, but pain one day and none the next can cause such havoc with your mental state.

One minute you feel better. The next minute you feel like you are starting over.

It's been 9 weeks with this wound–the wound I shouldn't have–and I am trying to maintain my focus on how far I have come. There is progress, I can see it myself, but the pain…

If I have to guess the lesson is that to appreciate what you have, you have to understand how hard things can be.

I know my suffering is minor compared to what others deal with when trying to fight cancer. I understand that my pain is not the worst pain.

But it is pain–and pain drains so much from the soul.

Just a few days ago I was told how much better I look and that I had some of my typical energy and flow about me. I love hearing that–it brings me hope that I am still here, in this very different body.

I need to remember those moments so that I can continue to make it through these moments.

Update on the plan is that I meet with radiation team in a few weeks–just to chat. I am still not convinced that I'm going to do radiation. Hormone suppression medication starts this weekend, and I am also able to enroll in a clinical trial if I wish. I still have to have my expanders removed and swapped out for implants, and then there is the ongoing wound which is still 16.5 cm long. Healing in other directions is apparent, but still look like someone tried to filet me.

Lots to do. Lots to deal with.

Christmas is a time for peace and joy. I plan to focus on that.

It was hard to focus on the positive steps forward, but I committed to that the prior month, so I want to honor what I had committed to. With the pain, I had to be patient, but pain was able to eliminate so much strength and focus.

That is why people become addicted to pain killers.

You just want the pain to stop.

The ongoing purpose of my life was not clear right then—I knew that I was here to be me. To do me.

I know that part of that was this journey, even with the pain and the suffering. I knew that I was to trust in my path, and to understand that the steps I took are the steps I was supposed to take.

But I have said it before, it is easy to get lost in the hard and difficult times.

I wanted others to take away from this journal a sense of ability, of drive and to find ones self, but if I had to be honest, right then, in those moments, I didn't even want to find myself. I wanted to fly off into the sky and find a soft cloud to sleep on in the sunshine and be left alone. No doctors, no people, no pain and no worry.

I just wanted to be.

Instead of getting to do that, I continued to take in the good, breathe out the bad.

Every day can have a list of the good things—you can ALWAYS come up with something, even when the day was filled with terrible and bad things.

Write them down now. I had mine.

I held them close so I knew that there was still good around me.

Each day I looked for few more. Just like the tiny steps. Or the pennies.

The small ones started to add up after a while. If I had been smart I would have written them down on a small piece of paper, folded them up, and put them in a small jar. Then on the days that things were not as easy, pulled them out and reminded myself of all the small great things that I took the time to write about—small snippets that would make me smile.

Chapter Thirteen

Please don't worry

December 11

Yes I am in pain.

Yes this has been ongoing.

Yes it can be scary.

But I am okay.

Today I hit my breaking point of pain and called the nurse. The wound vac is turned off and the pain has receded.

I have relief.

What this means is that although the wound vac has done a tremendous amount of healing for me, it may be time to change to a new plan. Every day pain is not good for healing, and that is where we have been now for quite some time.

I just wanted to reassure those that sent such kind notes and are so worried about me. It seems I am only writing about the bad and not the good, which is truly not how my spirit works.

But sometimes pain can paint the entire canvas of your life and you can't see anything else.

Time for me to get a new brush.

We will see what we can do to improve things. I trust my care team and they know when I say I'm done, I'm done.

And I'm done.

More to come–thank you all for the prayers and messages.

Short update

December 17

I am back in the ICU with a severe infection in one of my expanders. Not the original source but it jumped there. Sepsis twice in 6 weeks is hard on my body.

Living on massive antibiotics and fluid (took 5 Liters to get me stabilized) I am finally turning this around.

Thank you online shopping. And to those that have stepped in again to help on the home front. There will be some elves needed this week for sure–but first I have to bust out of here!

Take care and cherish every moment. Enjoy your holidays and time with friends and family! Lisa.

I am Free

December 29

It's true, in my own way, I am free.

Free of tubes, drains, PIC lines, wound vacs.

Free of something attached to me that was meant to keep me alive, help me get well, to make me heal.

Finally, I am free of monitoring something constantly to ensure it works correctly, flows, isn't clogged or doesn't leak. With the relief comes the reality of what I have lived through in the last 10 weeks, and how much my body has had to endure. I am not sure, when thinking back to this most recent ICU experience, how I did it. I know for sure that I did not do it alone.

I know you are out there, thinking of me, praying for me, ensuring that my family was taken care of—I know and my heart is full of your joy. I read my last post just today–not realizing that I had posted anything while I was in the hospital.

Apparently, that is how sick I was. Funny thing, I also ordered a lot of things from Amazon during that time, and spent the week before Christmas working on opening boxes of things that I had no memory of ordering. There are other things that happened during the hospital stay that I cannot remember–the pain of multiple IV attempts, CT scan contrast, entering the surgery suite once again, for the fourth time in 3 months.

But what I do remember is the heart of my doctors and nurses, the aides that cared for me, the family and friends that visited, and the staff that stole a moment to say hello and check in on me. I remember feeling terrible, maybe the worst in my life, and people constantly checking on me to ensure that I was doing as well as I could be doing. I have now been home for a week and a half, and my body certainly lets me know what it has been through. Endurance is not a word in my current vocabulary, and hearing doctors use words like "labs off the charts" and "septic shock, yeah you look pretty good right now" brings reality home. But like all things, time will continue on, and with each day, I expect things to get better. Truth be told, not every day is better, but I can always find something that is better about each day. Whether it is driving myself to an appointment, or braving completing two loads of laundry in one day, it is better.

Today, with no tubes attached, I did my first day of yoga in 6 months. It is an app online that allows you to tailor the program to your skill level, and I started at the absolute lowest level.

And it was hard. And exhausting. And felt like an incredibly long 10 minutes. Most of the time it was deep breathing, with a little trunk rotation and happy baby thrown in, and it was incredible how resistant my body was to the movements. It is going to take time, along with really incredible nutrition, to bring things back to my normal. And by nutrition I mean lots of protein, fruits, vegetables, and combinations like liver and Vitamin C.

My body needs all the help that it can get right now to continue to heal. I still have a large abdominal wound to heal, and appointments to attend–so many appointments. But I am visualizing health and healing, taken on the new super hero nomenclature UNIBOOB, and vow to not be back as an inpatient at my hospital until I have a scheduled admission to deal with some of my future surgeries, and not one day sooner.

It is going to take time, lots of time, to heal. I understand that–I am not patient, but I will do my part to make it happen, as I recognize so many of you have done so much to support me and my family.

I look forward as always to updating you on my recovery path, and to support those of you also fighting cancer at this time.

We have crossed paths for a reason, and I pray your journey is easier than mine.

Know I am with you, walking and praying for your health and healing as well.

Witness for the New Year and an Anniversary

January 1

The New Year is here for all of us—and tonight I am spending some time reflecting back on last year, and looking forward to what will come next.

The "funny" part about today is that it truly has multiple meanings for our family. Of course it is the new year, and we all plan to make things new, better, different and exciting. The kids stayed up late to watch the ball drop, and today thoughts turned to the end of Christmas break, and returning to the real world of soccer, school and homework.

Five years ago, the holiday weekend was just like this one—an extra day off before returning to school and work, a day that was expected to be relaxing and fun.

It didn't happen that way.

Instead, tonight, right after midnight, will be the five year anniversary of Frank's crash.

Five years.

It feels like forever and a flash at the same time—it feels like yesterday, and a lifetime ago. After the last year with such a huge focus on my own health, I feel that I have been given a glimpse into the world of what a fighter Frank was while he worked to recover from his brain injury.

Although I was with him every day, being on the other side of a life and death battle is very different—and it changes your perception of everything around you.

You see every day differently; moments are cherished, recognized, understood and lived. If you choose, peace can reign, when living without fear of the future, and knowing that life will carry you where you belong.

I believed it 100% when Frank got hurt, and I believe it again now while fighting to recover from breast cancer.

I was privileged to witness a man fight for his life, and I would expect nothing less from myself at this point. It is a choice to do everything that I can to fight back, and fighting back is what I am doing.

Tonight, at dinner, the boys, Frank and I talked about what happened five years ago. The boys reflected back about that morning when they woke up and I was not home. They asked new questions–who knew first? How did I get to the hospital? Did I beat the helicopter to the hospital?

It was interesting to see them reflect back, and to ask Dad questions.

It was also interesting for them to connect how hard this past year has been as well, and to see the resilience in them as they asked what month I told them about my cancer, and that it seems like the year has gone fast.

I wish they did not have to be so resilient all the time.

I welcome the next year and whatever it holds for us. I know, and hold on to the fact that we can, and will, focus on what is important, and do our best to look forward into our lives.

It can be done, regardless of what else comes into our lives.

We have lived looking forward, not back, for five years.

And we won't stop now.

Happy New Year everyone–tonight I say my thankful prayer that Frank lived.

Another year had gone by. Had I lived in a way that I was proud of? That was filled with the things that I wanted to do?

Obviously not the year I had planned. Definitely not the year I wanted. But it was a year full of new things and opportunity. Choices, options, focus and plans.

Not all of them mine or what I would have chosen for myself.

As I look back at that time it became apparent that I was learning the most about myself. My children. My life. Trying to figure out how to "do" life while being ill was confounding. How do you plan a birthday party, shop for school clothes, get an oil change, all while trying to not cry from pain?

People live with these realities every day—and people LIVE with these realities every day.

They live.

My job was to figure out how to live now, with all of the scary things that had changed so quickly. Just trying to stay focused on moving one foot in front of the other every day was enough to make me exhausted.

In trying to put myself back into that place, I found it hard to breathe.

And that makes sense—that feeling of complete overwhelming shock. Nowhere to turn except to face forward.

It was the only choice.

Facing big life fears, those that expected, and those that are unexpected, is what makes us learn. We learn how we face difficult decisions, how we adapt, change and grow from situations out of our control.

Within your day, you make decisions about small things continuously. In hard times, we make decisions too, but sometimes they are made quickly, without looking at all of the variables. They might not be our best decisions, but they are decisions.

We get to own them.

Each day of struggling to live offered me the chance to review how I was living. What I was doing to be better, to think better, to listen better.

At the end of the year, I found the ability to still look for answers, for options that would support a good day versus a bad day. I wanted the good ones, the good times.

I didn't always find them, but I searched them out.

I want you to listen to yourself the next time you are unhappy. Listen to the inner talking going on in your head. You know it happens, we all have that inner voice.

What is your inner voice telling you? Is it good things? Bad things? Lists of things?

What is important when listening to the inner voice is recognizing if it is doing you good, or doing you harm. The voices that we pay attention to have a huge impact on how we think, feel and engage in the world around us.

Imagine if the voice that we hear the most—our own—was the voice that spoke the most joy, the most encouragement, and was our number one supporter.

Imagine a life of that voice.

Finding Balance–Again

January 5

Finding balance is a daily struggle–do more, do less.
    Rest and move.
    Do and Don't.
    I am finding it hard to find a way to find the best balance between the need to rebuild my strength, and still allowing my body to heal.
    There is so much healing that has to happen before I am even back to any semblance of normal.
    I realized again today how far I have to go before I will have my body back to where I want it to be. I had another appointment at the hospital today that took me to a few different departments. As I was walking through the hospital I became winded, and my hips started to hurt. Such small things but it made me realize that my body has been through a lot.
    It needs rest along with movement.
    Walking and weight lifting are the recommended treatments–with the temperature today at 0 degrees I think I may just do a bit of walking in the house. I am enjoying the yoga and hope that I can continue to keep that practice active in my day, and soon, move to more than 10 minutes per day.
    Onward and upward, feeling like I am on the right path.
    Fingers crossed and prayers that everything will stay stable.

Carrying Wood

January 15

Today I carried wood.
 So what, right? Big deal Lisa, you carried some wood.
 Well, it is a big deal.
 For months, I have been "resting." Healing from so many surgeries, chemicals, medications and insults to my body. With rest also comes the reality of muscle wasting, and by now, my muscles have really deteriorated–muscles in places I bet you don't even think of, like your fingers.
 Yep, even my fingers hurt these days.
 Every day I try to do a little bit more of real life–laundry, driving, making food, picking up and taking care of myself. Each day I wake up sore and hurting, knowing my muscles are working hard to build back up, even while my body heals.
 It has been discouraging at times to see how truly weak I have become, like when I tried to put a 6 pack of pop back on the shelf, and I had to use two hands.
 It feels pathetic.
 I know, I am grateful to be alive, feeling better, and able to reclaim a little bit more of real life every day.
 Today, for the first time in 3 months, I was able to shower without plastic wrap taped to my body somewhere (I know, TMI, but for me, it was wonderful). No more fighting against the giant wound, PIC line or stitches—now the thing I fight against is this crazy curly hair.
 I was lucky enough to get to spend the weekend with my parents up north, doing a little baking, and sitting by the fire. It was relaxing and quiet and peaceful. The large fireplace is blissfully warm and

wonderful to sit near. But, having a fire all the time require wood. And wood doesn't walk inside by itself.

Normally there are kids around to move wood, but this time it is just me.

So if you want a fire, you get to move the wood.

I brought the carrier outside and loaded it with half the wood that I would normally load. I carried it into the house and piece by piece, moved it into the wood bin.

Then I had to sit down. I was tired already, but determined to at least get enough wood for an afternoon of fire.

Each day I brought in a little bit more—and each night my muscles reminded me that it had been a while since I had asked them to perform.

For me, moving wood felt like a triumph—a return to real life.

Add in a discharge from the wound nurse team, discharge from home care, and a return to work this week, and life looks pretty good.

Now to just make it through the upcoming five and a half weeks of radiation, and hopefully, eventually, get back to full-time work, and it will be great.

For now I will settle with part-time work, fewer doctor appointments, and continuing to get better.

Only looking forward now.

Looking back doesn't do anyone any good.

The Things I didn't know

January 22

There are so many things that I didn't know when diagnosed with breast cancer almost a year ago.

I didn't know that things would start so fast; the visits, the appointments, the doctors.

I didn't know how well acquainted I would become with needles–so many needles that I lost track. The more months that past, the more needles I knew, and with each time, the bite became a little bit worse.

I didn't know I would have 11 surgeries in a year–and that I would know anesthesiologists by name. Nurses, aides, housekeepers and nutrition staff all became my friends–and shook their heads, sad that I had returned to the hospital again, and again.

I didn't know I would lose friends–that people would walk away without a glance back. Scared, mad, frightened by the diagnoses? I will never know why.

I didn't know that I would face fear, anger, death and pain, coming at me from all sides, sometimes joined together.

I didn't know about the unrelenting pain.

I didn't know if I would live.

I didn't know about the friends I would make–those new people that filled my life with joy. Or the friends that would stay and brave the journey, and help to brace for the impact of each physical and emotional blow.

I didn't know I would gain perspective, and understand more about the strength that can grow from the depths of hell. Or how from the darkest days come the brightest light.

I didn't know how people would rally and support, lift up and carry my family for weeks on end. That those I knew a lot, and those I knew a little, would all make sure that my home was filled with unbreakable support and love.

I didn't know it would be so hard.

And I didn't know it would be so amazing.

There are so many things that I didn't know, and so many things that I am happy that I found out. And without breast cancer, I would never have known.

When we are seeing with more than just our eyes, the world opens up to immense joy and visions. During cancer, my eyes and my world were opened up to more than I could ever have imagined. I learned a new level of love, joy and feeling that I never knew existed in the world. I learned feelings so intense, brought to me by the smallest moments in time, that they engaged my heart like nothing else ever has. Envision the movie "The Grinch" when the Grinche's heart, so small and dark, grows three sizes in a day. My heart, never dark to begin with, exploded with light, and I was honored to be able to learn new lessons each day, brought on by breast cancer.

What I didn't know brought me the largest gifts—and an understanding of the world in so many new ways.

Chapter Fourteen

What's new?

February 19

What's new with all of you? I feel as if I haven't been a good writer lately. It isn't because things are going badly, on the contrary, things are moving along just nicely.

I have 14 of 30 radiation treatments completed.

I am working three days a week.

I am able to go to my son's soccer games.

I can drive to the lake house and visit my parents.

All good thing that I couldn't do a month ago–I keep telling people that things are certainly looking up. I am happy, feeling good and living my life.

Cancer is a part of my life, but it isn't everything in my life. I have other things to do than think about the things that exist because of cancer.

Rashes that itch.

Pain that is always present.

Tiredness.

Ridiculous hair.

Some things are just not as important as other things. The good and the fun are where energy is spent. Not on worrying about what might happen, what is currently happening, and why cancer is here.

Cancer does not get my energy. Radiation, doctor visits, labs and tests do not get my energy.

My energy is giving to the people in my life, both old and new. These days it feels like the new may outnumber the old friends. So many links to others, first through brain injury, and now through cancer.

Wouldn't it be great to have those connections to others without the traumatizing life events? Wouldn't we all be happier and healthier if we could connect with others in ways that were truly meaningful without being driven together by fear or uncertainty?

These days with technology and social media, I will admit it is much easier to "connect" with people without being in the same room. Even being an extreme introvert, I find that human connection means much more in person.

Cancer has taught me many things, and one of the best is that living life without true connections, even just a few, is lonely.

I hope that you can find a new connection this week–even one– to make a difference in your life.

Connecting the dots. Connecting the people. Connecting with others.

The key to happiness is connections.

Now I am not proclaiming this as the solution to all things, but I am going to continue to focus on ways to bring change.

In a way, the hard change of my past experiences brought the changes of new. Change in that sense is a good thing, change that came along with growth. And connections.

In the past I have noted that people often do not truly connect—as I stated in my post, it is easy to connect to others, to get things that we need, without even looking someone in the eyes. Technology, fast paced society, changes in social structure. All of these things have made it easy to avoid connections.

But is that the best way to live? Of course, speaking as an introvert, I relish in the reduction of actual connection. But let me tell you, when I am engaged enough to feel a true connection with someone, it is amazing.

Connections with others are often broken with illness and trauma. We are changed, the people around us are changed, and normal parts of life shift into different patterns—different connections. Some of these may not be what we want, but they exist because of the change.

Our job, our choice, is whether or not we want to accept the changes.

The new connections.

If you are faced with something new, something scary, you may also be facing new connections. My advice to you? Give them a try.

I am a firm believer that people are put in our paths for a reason. We may never know why, but be curious. Be engaged.

What can a new connection, even during a time of terrible struggle, mean to you?

I Quit

March 2

I quit.

Well, not today, but I quit yesterday. I know you are thinking that quitting sounds like a negative thing, but for me, it is truly joyous.

I quit radiation.

I was scheduled for 30 sessions of radiation–25 regular sessions, 5 days a week, and then 5 "bolus" sessions. I made it through 10 sessions before my skin started to react and by 17 my skin was on fire. Rash, red, angry itchy skin. We held radiation for a few days, tried new creams plus prednisone, and nothing worked.

A few days ago I was running the boys to soccer and friends and realized that my skin hurt. A lot.

I started talking to myself in my head as the boys were singing in the background in the car.

I literally asked myself why I was doing this. My skin HURT and I didn't like it. I wondered what would happen if I decided to stop.

To be done.

Right now.

The bliss that came to my heart when I had this thought was palpable. I could be done. No one was making me do this.

I could quit.

So I did. I walked in and told my nurse and doctor that I was done.

It was an amazing, freeing feeling.

I am happy to say that I am no longer facing weeks of more treatment. I am done. My body can spend the next few weeks healing. My heart and soul are calm and at peace with this decision.

I believe in medicine and the community of medical practice. I trust my doctors and their recommendation.

But I also trust that I know my body and I know what is best.

So I am done. I am heading in a different direction with the focus on rest, nutrition and healing. I still have two surgeries to go, but I will face them feeling confident with my health.

Cancer can just go away. There is no room for you here.

A letter to my best friend

March 13

I dreamed about you last night. It doesn't happen often, but last night we were back together again.

Although parts of the dream were fleeting, it warmed my heart this morning to know we spent a few more moments together, even if it was in the dream world.

In the beginning I didn't know you were there—I was in a college dorm hallway trying to get in line for a shower. Another friend of mine was in there, so I put my clothes and things down to wait. I went back a few minutes later and greeted her as she was leaving. I walked into the room and it was a very messy dorm room.

Clothes were strewn everywhere and I saw milk and some other groceries on the counter to put away. In my head I was laughing at the mess knowing you would never have allowed a room to look like this.

I opened the small dorm fridge and it was almost full but I started to cram stuff in. That was when you arrived and started laughing about how full the fridge was. We both started working on getting things put away as I slowly became aware of my alarm going off. I woke into a gradual understanding of my wakeful state and that I had been dreaming.

I was happy to see you again—there are few in this world that I connect to in the way that we did, although most of that connection for us was based on growing up together. The Lisa/Lisa partnership was a great one, and one that would have been lovely to carry into adulthood.

We didn't get that chance. Cancer abruptly interrupted the beginning of your grownup journey, and ended 10 years later. So many things we didn't get to experience together, so much time lost. But I wanted to thank you for some insight into your world. You have helped me live life differently, to appreciate so many things, and to take notice when I might otherwise lose sight of what is important.

See, I have cancer too. What are the odds? Although a different type of cancer than what you had, the diagnosis made me think of you. That initial fear and dread, the instant fight reflex, the shock and awe that takes over.

How could this happen? How did you cope? I remember the day you told me, I remember the crying, the disbelief.

I remember that I wasn't here for most of your journey. We were so young, only 21, and not even in the same state. We talked often, but it wasn't the same. I didn't get to go to your appointments, be with you when you woke up from surgery, hold your hand during the pain, or make you a meal. I could pretend it wasn't so bad when you brushed it off, told me you were okay, and we talked of other things. I wasn't here. I had my own life to live.

These days I am on your side, telling people that it is okay, fighting against the fatigue and the pain, thanking people for endless meals and support, and living my life. But I learned some very important lessons during your battle; I just didn't know I was learning them at the time.

Lessons that you didn't have as you braved cancer so much younger than I am now.

I've learned to always look for the good in every day, even the days filled with pain or tiredness.

I've learned that I cannot control everything, and trying to do so causes more damage than good. Trying to control everything causes more stress than relief.

I've learned that what my kids need from me is time. My time. Not clothes, or gifts, or things. Just me. As I am.

I've learned that relationships are everything. Even the hard ones.

I've learned that you were stronger than I ever knew.

And that your daughter is just like you.

I won't get to share with you how amazing it has been to watch her grow up, smiling like you. Smart. Beautiful.

And gracious.

I won't get to ask you how you did it–surviving, fighting, living with your pain, losing your vision, losing so much of who you felt you were.

But I know in my heart that you paved a way for me to be brave and to fight the battle differently, that your gift to me was courage. I'm sure you didn't know the gift you were giving. The gift you gave me even as you were dying.

But I know. I understand.

Thank you for showing me what you didn't know. For being my friend and my strength at a time when I didn't have much of either. For sharing with me all of you.

I miss you–it's been a long time. You come to mind when I don't expect it. Some times over and over for days, then nothing for months. Know that you build me up and bring me peace when I worry.

Thank you for being my best friend. Thank you for being an example of bravery.

Thank you for showing me the way.

You are missed. Your best friend, still here on earth.

I love you.

Lisabeth

It's just Cancer

March 29

The last few weeks have been a very slow return to what I see as semi-normal life.

The days are filled with work, soccer, school and errands. I usually make it through the beginning of the week, but by the end of the week, I am wiped out.

I hear that it is normal, and it will be like this for a long time.

A year.

So how does one concede to having a few good days, and then a few days that you want to just crawl into bed and stay there. Oh, and there isn't really much sleep involved, just sitting still, resting and spending a lot of middle of the night time on Pinterest.

Nothing is normal, nothing is abnormal.

Life is moving along as it always does, and I am doing my best to continue to live life.

You know why?

Because this is just cancer.

Cancer doesn't take over unless I let it.

Cancer doesn't get to be in control, unless I let it.

Cancer doesn't get to run my life, unless I let it.

So I don't. Many days I don't even remember I had cancer. Fatigue reminds me. Doctor appointments remind me. Pain reminds me.

But I don't live with cancer.

Cancer occasionally interrupts my life.

Thank you for asking, I am doing okay.

I go to work. I work out. I do fun things with my kids. I hang out with Frank.

I only look forward, I do not look back.

I spent last weekend in the ER with pain. But testing shows that it is nothing major, more likely an adhesion caused by all of the surgeries in my abdomen. Not fun but not a big deal.

Just another day in paradise.

I love having cancer

April 8

I love having cancer–I really do.

You know why? Because it truly puts everything into perspective.

I have spent over a year fighting, being sick, living with pain, surgeries, toxic medications and hospital visits, and I can honestly state that I am very happy.

This weekend I was lucky enough to spend five days in Memphis with my daughter and my mother. Now if you know anything about our lives, you understand that for both my Mom and I to leave town takes an act of Congress, flying my brother into town, and a lot of prayer that nothing will go wrong.

Well, lots of things did go wrong but none of it was vitally important.

What was important was the time spent with two of my favorite people. Although the trip had purpose—Mariah was presenting her research poster at an undergraduate research conference–the rest of the time was spent visiting gardens, hanging out and eating great food.

It was blissful.

And not once did I think about cancer.

Don't get me wrong, things still hurt, hot flashes suck and my hair gets more ridiculous by the day, but I just don't care that much.

This is my life–not cancers life–and I am living the way that I should be.

Full engaged. Having fun. Loving life.

Because that's what we should all do every day.

You can spend time worrying, or you can spend time living.

I choose living.

Sitting in the dark

April 23

I'm sitting here in a dark hotel room with my 12 year old son snuggled up to me.

It's quiet and I'm awake.

I'm always awake. But that's okay.

I'm thinking about how I wish I had spent more time walking or on the treadmill yesterday instead of playing Tiny Tower on my phone.

I tell myself that I can do it today–which is true.

I also tell myself that it's ridiculous that I made that choice. This pain is nothing compared to the pain that others endure. This pain isn't stopping me from doing things like going for a walk–it's the choices that I make that stop the walk/run/yoga from happening.

It's just pain.

I just get tired of it sometimes.

Figuring it out

April 28

After living the last year with a cancer diagnosis I am never surprised when things change.

The last few weeks have been different in that doing the daily day-to-day has become difficult.

There is the ongoing pain, mostly in the joints of my legs, knees and feet, although sometimes my shoulders and hands like to join in the fun.

There is new weight gain which is odd for me, which isn't helping the giant abdominal scar feel any better.

I'm constantly cold–so cold that I am not warm even with the heat in my car on high. I just don't feel real great.

I had my pre-op visit today–I don't see my GP very often since I have so many other doctors involved in my care.

Oncology. Gynecology oncology. Radiation.

Thankfully he knew me "before" and was actually the doctor that first called to tell me I had breast cancer. We talked about how I have been feeling and reviewed my recent labs. He decided to check them again, both of us hoping my white count would be normal.

All my labs were normal except for my thyroid, which is over double the normal number.

For me that is great news as it explains all of my symptoms, and eliminates any new real bad things. Hopefully an adjustment to my meds will fix all of this stuff so life can settle down before my surgery at the end of May.

Today just proved that although I do not let cancer run my life, it is still in the back of my mind. As I hear stories daily about others fighting for their lives I find it hard to complain about pain and feeling cruddy.

Every now and then I let a little whining loose.

I'm done now.

It is true that somewhere along the months of cancer, surgery, needles and pain there was a shift in who I was. I became the new me because the old me had to break through what life was handing out and arrive at a new place.

The new place was similar, in that the world didn't look too terribly different, but I was different.

The choices I made, from what to eat in the morning, to whom I spoke to, to how I engaged with the people around me, was different.

Others noticed, and asked about the level of calm that I presented. Now don't think I did not attribute some of the calmness to the fact that I was still living in recovery mode, and had a lot of healing left to do. But I also told people that at some point I had to let go of trying to make myself fit into what I perceived as the normal box of my world, and bend a bit to fit into the new one.

I am bendy. I can change. I made that choice.

I saw other during this time that had made different choices. Choices to stay in fight mode, denial mode, and I would never tell anyone that they were wrong in their choices. We get to make the choice as to how we will engage with our own lives.

What I recommend is that we pay attention to the life around us, and let some of what is around us guide the course. Now this does not mean that just because you saw the Garth Brooks tour bus on the highway that you should give up your entire life and job to go on tour and be a professional groupie. Not quite what I meant. But I do mean that by being a conscious part of the day, the day will guide you to somewhere you may not have meant to go.

A place that could enrich your life.

We just have to make the decision to do it.

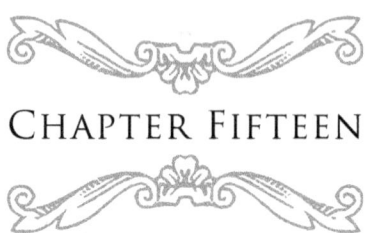

Chapter Fifteen

This thing called lymphedema

May 17

I know it's early.

    Sleep is often elusive in my world and I try to just rest when I find myself awake and alone at night. This morning I find myself awake and bored, so here I am again to bring you a glimpse into the cancer world.

    As I get closer to surgery next week I have found myself in more pain and with a new diagnosis.

    Lymphedema.

    Go google it. I'll wait.

    Got it? So here's how it works in my world. As I get dressed every day I "choose" to wear a medical prosthesis to equalize my breasts so that I can wear my work clothes and look symmetrical. What that really means is I wear a giant ugly bra with a super heavy "fake" boob in it so I feel more like myself.

    I've been noticing lately that it's more uncomfortable, and even t-shirts we're starting to bother me. I fuss with the left side, it feels tight, and my armpit is bothering me.

    I finally used my brain and asked an OT at work to check it out.

    And of course my left arm, the side that had surgery and was at risk for lymphedema, is larger than my right now.

It explains a lot; the soreness, the clothing that's too tight on that side, the constant feeling of it being "different".

So now I get to do more things in my day that focus me back to cancer and the aftermath.

Stupid cancer.

New massage/exercises and another "medical" device–compression garments.

Now these are not attractive, although they can be neutral and easy to hide.

But as you all know–hiding from this crap is not in my nature.

So instead, I followed the advice of my OT–who understands my passion for facing things head on–and went to a very cool website called LympheDIVAs.

Go check it out–I know you want to.

Amazing right?? If you have to wear compression garments you might as well make the statement that cancer doesn't win.

So I am patiently waiting for my first two sleeves to arrive in the mail, and I start OT today for a lesson in how to fight back from this new disruption on my life.

It's my choice–my choice to not just live with this new facet of my life, but to embrace it. I have found that embracing each part of this cancer journey makes living my life on my terms that much easier.

Yes–pain is constant. I choose to do as much as I can each day, including coaching soccer for my sons team, despite having to limit my activity.

Yes–I choose to have surgery again to replace the expander that was lost during the second round of infection last year. To me it is a means to end the giant bra problem and to get back on my original path of moving past cancer and back to my life.

Yes–I'm tired. The pain from the new meds has become unbearable, and I chose to stop taking them again. I will try a different one in a few weeks.

I guess all I have to say about lymphedema is that it's just another part of cancer that can enter your life.

I choose to embrace it and not let it define me, just as cancer does not define me.

27 Dresses–The Cancer version

May 21

27 Dresses–most of us have seen this movie or at least know what it's about.

A young lady is the caregiver to all, and has had that role for many years. In that time, she has been part of many happy events, mostly weddings, and with each one she purchased a bridesmaids dress.

As the story unfolds, her controlled world and space are invaded by two things–her younger sister, and a reporter, both of whom destroy her carefully organized life.

The reporter visits her home for an interview, and finds her hidden stash of bridesmaid dresses–each one with their own story. At first, she tentatively allows him to see her vulnerability by trying on one of the dresses.

Eventually she shows them all to him, relishing in the memories of each wedding. Events that she was a part of, but maybe not always present.

As her idea of truth of her life is pushed past her limits, she is forced to realize that being "part" of life doesn't mean just doing as many things as possible, or organizing the world.

It is the moments that are important.

Paying attention and living in each one, and not being focused on the tasks at hand. Engaged memories mean so much more than the selfies we take, the Snaps we send, or the posts we "like" on Facebook.

Life is meant to be lived–none of us know how much life we truly have.

I became aware just today of a path that I am following—a realization that I have already accepted, but maybe didn't realize it was now the center of my life.

Dresses.

What about the dresses you ask?

Well, since my surgical mishap in the fall and the subsequent giant scar on my belly, I cannot wear pants. I spent the winter wearing fleece leggings, skirts and shirts. Comfy for sure, cute at times, but nothing that I can wear in the summer.

Historically I have not been a fan of dresses. I'm not much of a "girlie-girl" and I hate shopping.

But lately I have been finding myself drawn to more and more dresses. Bright colors, some short, some long, but all extra fun.

You see, it will be months before I can wear pants that do not have the word "yoga" in front of them. So why not embrace this time and go all out—and buy dresses.

So I do.

At least one a week.

I admit I had a dress "moment" two weeks ago and bought five. Yikes.

But what's great is that I LOVE them!! With each one I can remember why I loved it, where I bought it from, and how it made me feel.

My 27 dresses will be part of moments that I choose to live in.

Facebook has become my own personal dress show—yes I am a firm believer that Facebook knows all, and it shows me new dresses every day.

For me the moments matter.

I will spend this time feeling good and (hopefully) looking good as well.

Wearing my many dresses in comfort.

Now shoes. That may be a problem.

I still hate shoes.

It will be okay

May 23

I know you are worried.
    I know you are scared.
    But it will be okay.
    I love the hugs, the good lucks and the prayers. Each one warms my heart.
    The "Mom you scare me with these surgeries" are more real in their expression of fear.
    But it's going to be okay.
    We can't spend our time thinking about what might happen.
    Let's think about what we are doing this weekend, what flowers still need to be planted, and what kind of cookies we should bake.
    So let's not worry about surgery tomorrow. Tomorrow is just another day.

So far so good

May 30

I hesitate to post that things are okay as that has often been about the time when things go bad.

I decided to risk it and say that I am doing well.

I spent the last week recovering at my parent's house. I figured staying at home and attempting to rest would result in me working on projects.

I don't sit still well.

So sitting at the lake and watching the birds was a good choice. It also helped that the weather has been crummy.

I head home tomorrow to a doctor appointment and hopefully a little bit of planting.

I'm taking it easy. I'm resting. I'm trying to sleep.

Thank you for thinking of me–I appreciate your prayers and well wishes.

Let's say it is going well.

Moving on–Part 6

June 3

It is time to move on.

I am lying in bed wishing I was asleep. The sun is shining right in my face which makes sleep elusive. But to me, sunshine is a healing joy, and I really don't need sleep right now. I'll enjoy the sunshine instead.

I went to the doctor yesterday and was cleared to return to work next week. I didn't expect anything less. This wasn't a major procedure and there should be a good outcome.

But you never know.

Even with all of the drama and fear associated with the last year of cancer treatment and emergency surgeries and procedures, I have not lost my optimistic internal clock. Those around me seem to worry so much more than I ever do–worry was something I gave up a long time ago when I embraced the understanding that I have very little control of anything other than myself.

I learned that how I react to life around me is fully within my control.

The rest? Not so much.

Giving up control (the control I never truly had anyway) was the hardest and easiest thing I have ever done.

Being at ease with my life allows me to look ahead and move on with life in a much more purposeful way than before. Yes, I still have a surgery looming in the fall. Yes, there are still many doctor visits in my future. Yes, pain is probably going to stick around for a while.

But as I said before, I get to control how I face and react to all of these parts of my life.

So I chose to move on. Move on with life plans, summer plans, kid plans and family plans.

There will be interruptions I am sure, but bringing my center back to health and life will only improve my mental health and well-being.

And that's always been the goal.

Moving on now. Going to stay here and hang out in my sun puddle for a bit.

Then it's time to find my gardens.

Boobs 2.0

June 7

So boobs. Yep let's talk about boobs.

So I'm trying to get mine back–a newer maybe slightly younger looking version than before. As part of that there are several surgeries.

Putting things in.

Inflate.

Remove and replace.

You get the picture.

The goal is to be able to feel comfortable in my own skin and my old clothes. That is why I chose to go forward with this type of reconstruction.

Last weekend while I was "resting" I pulled a muscle in my chest. I know you are all yelling at me for not resting. But I wasn't doing anything at that time to hurt myself.

I was putting on my seatbelt.

So dumb.

Anyway, my chest was still bothering me on Monday so I went to see the surgeon. Because of my history, they felt it best to have an ultrasound and a needle aspiration of the fluid that was now collecting near my new expander.

Can't seem to escape these procedures involving needles.

Procedure was a bit nerve racking but simple enough. He pulled 80cc of what the doctor referred to as "old surgical blood" out of the site, and today it is sore but probably on the way to healing.

Fun time as always.

Now if I could only lift my arm above my head again I would be Golden!!!

Soon enough....

Can't stop now

June 21

Things have been going well with just a little process issues. What this means is that every few days I had to have blood drained out of the expander site. Nothing to worry about, I just needed to be diligent about getting to my appointments.

Yesterday I went for a walk with a colleague during lunch. As we walked back into the hospital I joked with her about my left chest area felt like I was having a contraction. It kept going for a few more minutes and I decided to check it out in the mirror.

My breast had doubled in size, and was continuing to grow.

Very quickly I ended up in the ER and they called a rapid response (code for hurry up and get into this room).

My breast kept getting bigger and tighter and more painful. Apparently I had a hematoma around my expander.

We all agreed that emergency surgery was on the agenda.

So off I went back to surgery–not what I had planned for my afternoon.

So I am home, back in bed, and super irritated by this latest drama.

There is a positive in that I did get to keep my expander.

The hard part is we are supposed to leave for Chicago on Thursday for a soccer tournament.

Now what....

Impatient

June 27

I'm sitting and waiting for Frank to fly in to Chicago so he can help me drive back from a very long weekend of soccer and a work conference.

Normally I would jump in the car and go, but my body just will not allow it.

My brain is feeling betrayed by the abilities of my body.

Bored but can't move.

Tired but not tired.

Engaged yet frozen.

I have never been more frustrated than I am right now. At least when I was critically ill I felt terrible–I didn't want to do anything even if I could.

Now, I want to do things but my body says no.

This is NOT how I live my life.

#cancersucks #getoutofmyway

Does it ever feel like no matter what you do to move forward that something keeps pulling you backwards?

I was astounded that I could even see four feet in front of me somedays when I felt like I was just getting shoved back by a wind storm. The hits kept coming, the problems kept coming, and there really wasn't anything that I could do about any of it other than make the decision to get up again the next day and take steps to the next thing.

I knew that I was getting better, feeling better, because I was getting more crabby and bored. Unhappy with the rate of healing, and unhappy with the setbacks that kept arising. So little control over my own life.

And yet, I kept writing about how to find small joys, different views of the same world. Finding things that made me happy even when I wasn't happy.

I am a believer that we can change the direction of our own lives. It takes patience and focus. It takes commitment and a plan. It does not, however, take a huge amount of change. It can be a small thing, a small decision that makes all of the difference.

I believed all of the advice I gave, and struggled to take it myself. Some days I could truly embrace being me, and others, I just wanted it all to end, a do-over, to go back to the way things were.

Not surprising, but interesting to read in hindsight.

Humans, in general, want to feel good, do good, and be good. Fairly simple, unless you add in the push and pull of the world around us, and then it might not be so good. But good is as relative as anything else we measure the world, by, so how do we measure happiness? Contentment? Where is the barometer for goodness?

It is all up to us, our reactions to the swirl around us. We decide. I decided. You decide.

Apparently I decided to be mad at cancer and struggle with my inner battle of doing versus being for a while.

And that's okay. It was my decision.

Chapter Sixteen

Thinking about tomorrow

July 16

Typically I will start my posts with some pithy commentary relating to my title. I start out with something sassy and build from there.

Today I'll I've got is that–thinking about tomorrow.

See, tomorrow is scan day. Tuesday is results day. Not fun words for anyone that has been diagnosed with cancer.

I don't spend time worrying, but I will admit that I have been thinking about it. Wondering if I'm headed back to chemo. More surgery. Added pain.

As a positive thinker I promise I am not dwelling on it–but it's out there today.

How much more can one take? I'm not sure there is an end, I think we as individuals can take and do much more than we think we can. It's just easy to get wrapped up in the hard stuff.

I'm going to get going with my day–one son dropped off at his sisters, another headed to soccer, the third to work. I'm going to sit in my garden for a moment and appreciate the beauty of the morning.

And then move on.

It's what we do–survivors–we just move on.

Moving on

July 18

Great news today–clean CT scan which means no current cancer in sight.

With this news, I officially move on from the cancer fight. I know that it can return.

I am a realist.

But I will not let it direct or rule my life.

The new question is the pain. My oncologist does not know why I have so much pain still–we are going to try a few things to see if my body is fighting against itself after being assaulted by so many surgeries, drugs and antibiotics in the last year.

Hopefully we can figure it out.

Pain is exhausting.

Tomorrow is my new normal.

More of the good

August 2

I am happy to report that the good news keeps on coming. Today I met with my plastic surgeon to discuss the plan for surgery this fall. I have been preparing myself for another long recovery period since the initial conversations involved some major repair of this giant wound scar along with completing reconstruction.

When we chatted today she checked out the abdominal canyon I call this scar, and since it has healed so well (well, being a relative term I assure you, only she can say that and me not want to punch her) my recovery down time could be as little as 5 DAYS!!

5 DAYS- are you kidding me?? In my world that's like 15 minutes. As long as I can stay out of the Emergency Room and have no more sidebar surgeries or infections I am on my way to a short stay.

The joy this brings me is almost immeasurable. To get to a point that I only need a small amount of time off and then to get back to life is almost too good to be true.

It doesn't mean I get to go jumping back to working out. But even two weeks is significantly less than the 8-12 days off that I was planning on.

Hear that sound? It's the sigh of relief I just let out. I think I have been holding my breath for too long.

Happy One Year

August 11

I am happy to be one year out from chemo. Chemo was incredibly hard–people that endure chemo are reborn on the other side.

A different person emerges from the ashes of chemo.

Thank you for staying with me during this year. It means everything to have my village.

Sometimes living your life while dying can be the best life ever.

Missed it

August 26

I completely missed it—I did not write a blog, or a note or anything at all last week, even after hanging out in the hospital for three days. Apparently they didn't count!

Although not as serious as my other hospital stays, I had another round of IV antibiotics before a surgery to replace one of the expanders with an implant. Not on the agenda for last week but my agenda is often replaced with the bigger life agenda.

It felt odd being in the hospital without feeling terrible- a blessing for sure not to be fighting for my life.

Instead, I had some interesting experiences, like an IV in my neck, and a lot of great care from kind people.

I'm glad to be home. Now I just need to figure out this whole "resting" dilemma.

I'm exhausted yet life goes on–still working on balancing that somehow.

Only posting the good

September 21

I find that I post less when I am feeling better.

I find that I do not want to share only negative, so I only post the more positive.

Today I find myself back in the hospital, with another infection, and wondering how I ended up here.

Truthfully I KNOW how I ended up here–I went to see oncology because of some new pain on my chest wall, which needed to be checked out. But when checking that out, they noticed I had cellulitis brewing again on my left breast, and just like that, I am back on IV antibiotics.

Although tired, I feel fine, just a bit pucky from the IV meds.

I preach that life is meant to be lived, not survived. When we live our life, we are engaged, curious, excited and intentional. I work every day to live that life.

Today is no different. I feel good, I am working (a few floors higher than my office) and I will be back tomorrow.

That does not mean that I am not frustrated, sad and worried. Why these infections? Why is my body not doing what I want it to do? What is the new pain? How long can I deal with the chronic pain without having to add pain medication?

Today is another wonderful day–it is sunny and warm, and I plan to get out of here tonight and go watch another soccer game. Today I am upright, able to do some of the things that make my day complete, and I am hopeful for tomorrow.

Thank you for your prayers and messages. I will be fine.

Anyone keeping track of the number of surgeries, hospital visits and infections in this plot line? No? Truly I didn't either, until someone asked. At that time I had already had 14 surgical procedures, countless antibiotics and uncountable doctor visits.

Now I could have ticked them off, marking each one down like a badge of honor for passing by another milestone in this journey, but for me, it was not about how many procedures or appointments I could survive, it was about being present in them, and trying to learn how each one made an impact on my life. And impact they sure did.

I spoke earlier about the connections made, the paths forged, and I continue to believe that each person I encountered, each new face either with or without cancer, had meaning. I learned small things from people, things like they grew up a few blocks from where I did, or we both had the same English teacher in high school, and these connections brought with it that moment of smile, of happiness, that I would not have had, if it had not happened.

Those are gifts. Those small precious pieces of life should not be ignored.

But how to weave them into normal day life. How do we find a way to honor them when we are back and embracing life along a more typical path?

I do not have those answers yet. Even months later I still work to find a way to embrace the health along with the past illness.

Connections again.

Chapter Seventeen

The next big thing

October 7

Yesterday brought me within one week of what is supposed to be the final surgery for reconstruction. I, of course, am not counting on it being the last as we all know I tend the follow the path of MOST resistance these days.

However, next Friday I will head back to the hospital so that my plastic surgeon can finish my breast reconstruction. After that, she and another surgeon will tackle the huge abdominal scar that is my souvenir from that scary bowel perforation that occurred almost exactly a year ago.

When I met with the second surgeon this week he showed me the CT scan of my abdomen that clearly reveals that my abdominal muscles are not attached to one another; explains why I can't do much physically without feeling like I have to compensate with different muscles. His plan is to cut out the huge scar (5 x 20 cm) bring my muscles back to midline (which may require cutting smaller muscles on the side of my abdomen) injecting me with long acting pain meds, and sewing everything back up.

Sounds complicated. Sounds painful.

That is correct on both accounts.

Apparently the first few days aren't too bad, but once some of the meds wear off, it's going to hurt.

For about 6 weeks.

The good news is that the first week is the worst. And I can go back to work after the 2-3 week.

As he told me, "it's not as if you can tear anything, you will be rock solid when this is done. It will look great."

So the downside is more pain. I don't take pain meds–although I have a feeling I will bend that rule next week.

They understand (my care team) that I've been addicted to oxy once (another gift from the bowel perf last year) and that I would rather be in pain than take meds. Major surgery will make me adjust my thinking on that, but not for long. Pain is our body's way of making us pay attention. Pain is important and nowhere in healthcare does it say "I'm going to cut you open, resection your body, add some things, take something, see you back up and you won't have any pain at all!"

This expectation is why we have an opioid crisis in this country–pain is part of life.

Trust me I know. I live with it every day.

My plan–surgery Friday. Home Thursday. Rest. Rest. Follow up. Back to work the first week in November.

Seems like a great plan to me.

Now let's make it happen.

Truth

October 10

It's 0430 and I'm awake. I slept fairly well last night, which means I only woke up twice before drifting back to sleep. By 0430 I knew my luck had past and I started reading the news updates on my phone.

Its hard reading stories of such sadness like the one about a local paramedic killed in a crash last night. My heart hurts for that family and the world of first responders. But even as sad as it was, sometimes I feel like my heart has become so walled in that I don't feel some of the more impactful emotions.

I hate crying. It gives me a headache and makes me feel physically ill. Now I have it on good authority that crying should be a release of toxic emotions that frees our mind and body from those pent up emotions.

For some reason that just doesn't seem to happen with me. I wonder if it is because I hold myself and my emotions pretty close to my chest, a trick I learned after Frank got hurt to ensure that I didn't lose myself in the terrible fear of that time. The kids needed me, so I held it together.

I'm not sure that "skill" is serving me well.

I finally gave up and got in the bathtub. I spend a lot of time here each day, it is one of the few things that seems to ease the chronic pain that just keeps creeping through my body.

Warm water. Epsom salts.

Great healing combination.

I did a Facebook perusal while soaking and actually watched some of the videos that my friends had posted. I clicked on a video that I have scrolled by in the past.

It was about wrestler John Cena, who was being filmed opening thank you letters from his fans. They each talked about his mantra "Never Give Up". This video, this wrestler, is what finally brought me to tears today. He holds firmly in his beliefs that never quitting can bring you places that you never dreamed. Never quitting doesn't mean that bad things won't happen, but it's how you respond to those things that makes the difference.

Never quitting means don't lose hope.

I'm not a quitter. But I'm tired. And I'm in pain. And I just want the rollercoaster to let me off the ride so I can sit still for just a moment.

But that's not my journey right now. My journey is to leap forward to the end of the week and get through this next big surgery. It is necessary, just scary.

Some small part of me feels that if I can continue to take on this fight that somewhere, someone else has been given a pass. That they won't have to endure what my body has gone through.

I believe in the Universe. And I hope that someone is smiling and happy.

I will always carry the load for someone else.

Namaste

Pain-1 Lisa-0

October 17

Tough night. Pain is expected, even welcomed at some level, because pain is part of the recovery process. No one has a complicated abdominal surgery and reconstruction without pain.

It's the uncontrolled pain that makes it tough.

Last night I lived in a large pond of pain, and it took hours of changing and shifting to break the bubble and get my body to relax. An entire new process has been put into place to manage the pain differently, but with this gift comes the addition of another day here in the hospital.

For me, a minor loss.

I will miss AJ's big soccer game tonight. But leaving today is not an option if I want to get myself out of this giant canyon of pain.

Delays happen. I just am anxious to get moving with my life.

Praying for my body to brave the storm coming.

We are a team—my body and my souls—we just need to stay on the same page.

Pain-1 Lisa-1

October 18

Some gains in my world tonight. Pain has been controlled since mid-morning which means we may have figured out how to get through this tough healing process. With this gain comes the side effect of sleep. Sleep for me is always fitful–rarely do I sleep longer than 2-3 hours before waking up, sitting restless for a while before falling back to sleep. Late morning brought several medications to help stop the muscle spasms and relieve pain which made me groggy, and I slept for three hours.

I slept so hard I thought it evening when I woke up.

We kept the pain at bay most of the day which included another long nap in the afternoon.

I did not realize how little sleep I actually get every day until I finally got some solid blocks of sleep.

Pain is still well-controlled and I'm headed back to sleep.

If things stay stable I will get home today–and Home is where I want to be.

New twist

October 22

I now understand why people say to me "can't you just catch a break?"

Typically when friends and family are upset about some other hurdle or sideways path that pops up I just shrug my shoulders and move on. Everybody is different and heals in its own way. Sometimes the path to getting better is paved with some bumps and I react to them like I do to most things—let's get it dealt with and move on.

Today however, I official join the WTH club. Yesterday I finally caved and went to urgent care. I had been having increased pain in my arm all week and it had kept me up all night on Friday. It was this unrelenting pain that had significantly reduced my ability to do anything functional with my right hand. And it brought me to tears, which never happens.

After a long visit and an ultrasound, they found a blood clot in my arm near the elbow. And that is what is causing all of my pain.

Seriously. A blood clot.

Now this isn't one of the big scary blood clots that can kill you, which is a DVT. This is a superficial blood clot that is just making me miserable.

So now I get to take blood thinners for 6 weeks. The pain (supposedly) will gradually subside and that should be the end of it.

WTH. That's all I have to say.

Enough is enough.

Funny—my surgical incisions don't hurt at all. Instead I get to take tons of pain meds for this arm.

Enough already.

Another look into the world of ongoing sideline sitting.

Another block of writing focused on plans and patience, but can you also feel the impatience?

Inaction is in itself a form of action—one in which we have no movement but still may focus on the lack of movement. The brain does not want to rest, and the body is in need of peace and quiet.

How does one reconcile that? I am not so sure that is possible. I tried. It did not appear to go as well as I had hoped.

I knew at that time that I was writing to purge the thoughts of what I wanted to get done, so that maybe my brain would give me some peace and quiet while I was waiting out the healing part. But that was the point, waiting it out—waiting to jump back into life.

So, had I learned anything? Did I understand that as I said I wanted to learn from this experience, I write about the experience, am I really getting the experience?

As I look back, it appears that I did truly see the better in the world, even if I was viewing the world from the inside of a hospital. I found laughter with the nurses, I found a smile with the housekeeping team, and I wrote whenever I could. I tried to do things in a way that I felt would bring me to a place that as more positive than focusing on what had gone wrong now.

Squatting in the unhappiness would have been so easy. It was tempting.

I didn't choose that path. I cried. I was scared, and unhappy at times. I worried about the future. But then I sat in the minutes, the seconds, and knew that it would be okay. This was just another minute in time, a second of a day, and pain is not forever.

It may feel like pain is forever, but I have found that in the long run, you can even live with chronic pain.

It just is part of things sometimes.

So I ask you this, what does this all mean for YOUR life? How does any of this apply to you? In my heart I want everyone to be doing their best, living peacefully, energetic in their pursuits and their joys, not fighting with traffic, insurance bills or plumbers. I want people to pay attention and to be happy.

It must mean today that I feel that it is all about me—funny, I do not remember that being the plan for the universe, but there you go.

What do you want for you today?

Chapter Eighteen

My reality vs real reality

November 9

For someone that wants to be done with all things surgery and doctor related, a week with three doctors appointments and a call from the surgeon does not feel like things are done.

What was interesting is that now that my head is above water I have to think about things like the eye doctor, and maybe even a visit to the dentist. Because really, who has time for that when you are constantly in recovery mode?!

The surgeon call was a worry call on my part. This week has been marked by the right side of my abdomen feeling like it is being pinched in a large vice. Sometimes it feels too tight to even stand up, and to me it appears that there are even pockets of swelling. Since I stopped all pain meds (and blood thinners, woohoo on that one) I was starting to get worried about another famous Lisa Mackall complication.

Thankfully my surgeon put me at ease. Apparently the large internal stitches are most likely hanging out on a nerve, and they take 2 Months to dissolve. He asked how far post I was now and I told him three and a half weeks.

His response "And you're at work already huh?"

I laughed. Of course I'm at work.

This type of abdominal surgery takes a few months to quiet down and fully recover. He was not concerned about any of my symptoms, so neither am I.

Moving on.

Blood clot is healing well, the nerve pain is gone, but the weakness in my thumb continues. No clear answer on that yet.

So as it stands, all things are moving in a good direction.

Still tired. Now that I am off the pain meds for the blood clot the tendon pain is returning. Hair is longer. Still wearing scrubs most of the time so my abdominal skin doesn't hurt.

All in all improvements.

As for cancer, no sign at the moment. Scan again in February and the plan is it will be fine.

It better be. I have a date with the gym January 1 and cancer will not be breaking us up in 2018.

Beginning again

November 30

It feels like forever since I wrote an update. It isn't because there is nothing to write (there is always something to write) but I have been very focused on life and living.

There was a time that I wasn't sure how much life I had left. We all realize on some level that a new day is not guaranteed. Some of us have faced the reality that our last days may be sooner than we expect. During those times we can freak out or we can immerse ourselves in the joy and experiences that we have left.

I learned in that time that each day is a gift, and being well is an extra special gift.

I am working with a wellness coach and a physical therapist to recalibrate my body and my soul—recalibrate in the sense that if you become hyper vigilant to all the things that can and do go wrong with yourself, you fundamentally change the way your body works.

For me this has led to significant chronic pain.

When it came time for my last surgery in October, I was looking forward to it for two reasons. One, to repair my abdominal incision and muscles, plus finish my breast reconstruction, but also because I knew I would be back on pain meds that would eliminate my chronic pain.

And they did. That is the gift of opioids.

But as many of you know, after the scary near death experiences last fall and the subsequent open abdominal healing drama, I became addicted to opioids.

I will never forget the actual moment that I realized it. I couldn't believe it. Lucky for me I just stopped taking them in that exact moment.

Was it easy. No. Did I feel bad? Have pain? Yes, I did.

But I told myself no amount of pain was worth that slippery slope.

You see I work for an organization that openly talks about opioid abuse and the epidemic it is causing. I vividly remember a presentation from one of our leading physicians about how opioids change the way our brains work around pain. Our medical director spoke so passionately and openly about how patients can and do change the way their brains respond to the want of opioids, but it is a difficult process that so many people just cannot find their way through.

I told myself enough is enough–sepsis didn't kill me.

Opioids don't have a chance.

After my last surgery I was on opioids. And ALL of my pain was gone. It was a relief to wake up and not have to live with it.

But it was a short reprieve. I knew it was only a short break.

Because I stopped taking them after a few days.

Pain is back, but I don't believe pain is here to stay. My brain is sending messages to my body that have ratcheted up my alert responses. Essentially my "fight or flight" response is at red alert all the time.

Hence the pain, even when there is no reason for there to be pain.

This week I started physical therapy to begin the recovery that I want.

Bringing my body back to baseline. Increasing strength. Improving flexibility.

And decreasing the pain.

This will be a long slow process but it will happen.

Every day just a little bit more.

And someday I will wake up and realize that the pain will be gone.

I look forward to that day.

A few minutes alone

December 8

I am spending a few minutes alone.

In my car.

It's just about the only spot I am alone these days.

It's quiet other than the Christmas music playing.

Well, there are car doors slamming. And the kids running by with their soccer gear and hockey bags.

And some parents telling their kids to hurry up.

But other than that it's pretty nice.

Warm. Calm. Peaceful.

This time of year can be both wonderful and disheartening.

To some the holidays represent joy and wonder. Fun and love. Excitement and enchantment.

For others the holidays bring sadness. Sorrow. Heartache.

Last year at this time I was vacillating between being sick and being REALLY sick.

The holidays became unpredictable and painful for my entire family. We all worried about the next day. The next scare. The next infection.

This year is different for our family–but not for others.

There are other families that are spending this holiday season worrying about those around them that are ill, injured or, facing the most difficult times, passing from this place to another.

Those families need to know that we don't forget them just because our families and loved ones are well. We are the lucky ones right now–living our lives looking forward, enjoying the holiday season without the overlying fear of illness.

Don't forget those around you dealing with hard times. And if you have moved from the hard times, don't forget them.

Sometimes we learn the most, and love better, after the hardest and scariest times in our lives.

Thinking about it all

December 23

I pride myself on being able to look at my situation and my life in a positive way. I don't wallow in the scary mud of the difficult times that I have been through- I look for the moments, both large and small, that were the good.

There is always good.

Sometimes life brings us great news like a new baby or a promotion.

Sometimes we learn that a loved one has passed.

Each of these moments has the potential to bring change, and it is how you decide to hold it in your heart that makes a difference.

I saw one of my favorite doctors at work many times the last few days during our survey. He asked me several times how I was "really" doing.

My answer was always "great!"

Which is the truth. I haven't felt this good in almost two years.

I have energy to do the things I want to do during the day.

I am able to go to events and work without limiting myself.

I can immerse myself in home and work projects.

I am working out again.

I have started writing again and hope to publish another book next year.

And I'm currently cancer free.

All great things. All wonderful things.

That is the focus of my life. Of my day. In my heart.

But if I chose to, I could focus on the difficult things that still exist in my day to day life.

I am taking large doses of prednisone for a month which makes sleeping difficult

The pain–my daily companion- is always with me.

My workouts consist of band exercises and trying to get strong enough that it doesn't take a minute to get off of the floor.

I am still carrying an extra 15 lbs. from being sick which means I can't wear most of my clothes.

And even if I don't worry all the time, knowing I have scan in five weeks makes you wonder if cancer is hiding somewhere.

With all of that, I choose to find the sunshine every day.

It's possible. It's work.

But you can do it. Darkness doesn't have to be complete. When you find the light flickering in the dark, move towards it.

The light, however small, can sustain you even in the blackest of times.

Find your light.

Another year in the books, or should I say for this book?

I looked back at the last year of writing, comments and focus of where I have been. It has been a year of great chaos that I tried to focus into times of peace.

I believe that we are all part of this world for a reason—whether our time to engage with others is short or long, we are all given some time.

What we choose to do with it is of our own making.

I realized early on that writing frees me from worry. Writing gives me peace, and a place where I can lay down the scary and worry emotions onto paper, and then I let them go, free to touch other people.

Now I could see how putting my emotions out there can be seen as self-serving, a bit selfish even, but for me, there was never any expectation for others to read what I wrote down. Ultimately, the goal has always been to let people know how I was doing, and that I was okay.

Along the way I got a bit wordy, and in doing so, I hope that I helped another that may be crossing some of the same paths that I have been on lately. I wanted others to feel the connection, that others understand, and sometimes that understanding is all that we have to take us through the day.

As a society we often live inside our heads, along with social media, and we do not connect ourselves directly to others. Now I am a firm believer in writing to others, connection on Facebook or other forms of media, in fact bloggers have a great way of connecting to people. But I also encouraged the human connection, the touch, which conveys so much more than just words and warmth.

The connection between two people, even in the form of a hug or a handshake, can impact us on multiple levels far beyond the mind. In fact, in my past when I was not able to make that physical connection with my partner, I sought out a massage just to connect with another person.

Please do not take my idea of touch as permission to become a rogue hugger in the subway, but a chance to be someone that shakes hands firmly, gives a hug to others, and understands the meaning of human contact.

We, as people, need one another.

We need each other's ideas, comfort and emotion.

We need to be part of each other's lives, in ways that are meaningful, not superficial.

We need to connect. And then we need to notice the connections.

Not worrying about worrying

January 6

I don't worry. I don't fret.

But I do think about the future, and the time has come again for the future to be a bit worrisome.

Every six months people that live in the cancer world are brought face to face with the "what if."

The six month scan.

The first week of February I am faced again with a full body scan that will be looking for hidden cancer.

The same cancer that brought a two year journey of self-learning and pain.

When I say I'm not worried, I feel that my statement rings with truth, but I would be lying if I didn't admit to a few notes of fear sprinkled into these thoughts.

How can one be diagnosed with Stage IV cancer, survive treatment, and not wonder if something else isn't lurking behind door number two?

You can't.

Don't be concerned my friends–I am okay. I know the risks and I make many choices every single day that support my plan to live a long healthy life.

Lots of fruits and vegetables.

Reduced sugar.

Decreased stress with meditation, essential oils, deep breathing and quiet.

Exercise every day.

Eliminating chemicals in my environment.

Believing that facing my death has allowed me to now live my best life.

Whatever may be, I know that today, every day, I am living my best life with love and joy.

I am only looking forward, with lots of plans and fun on my agenda.

That is my plan.

The "Eve" of things

February 6

Last Saturday we were having our typical busy weekend. In the midst of it all Tommy declared the day Super Bowl Eve.

Technically he was correct and with all of the hype it felt like a special day.

Funny how the build up to things is sometimes almost as big as the actual day.

For me, tonight is CT scan Eve. Not nearly as fun or exciting, but just as stressful.

I could tell you that I am 100% certain it will be fine and I am completely chill about the whole thing.

But that would be a lie.

I am not worried. I am more uncertain that I want to do this again, and certainly not ready to hear that cancer is back.

I am preparing for good news–good news means another 6 months of just living and not worrying.

That's my plan and I'm sticking to it.

I'm lucky

February 8

I'm lucky–for so many reasons.

    I have amazing support in my life.
    I have a strong family, a strong will and a strong heart.
    I have people that will stand by me no matter what.
    I have a great job.
    I have great doctors.
    And today I got great news.
    A clean scan means more time without fear.
    It means I can do anything with less fear casting a shadow on my light.
    But it's never over.
    Luck is just that, and it can change at any moment.
    It's why I choose to be, at all times, living out loud. Living a life of engagement, of purpose–a life that I know, when I face death, that I won't regret.
    I don't need to think of death and worry that I didn't live life.
    Facing death last year made me realize that I need to ALWAYS live my best life.
    Don't let it take death to make you live yours.
    Grateful for my good news today.
    Blessed to be able to face tomorrow.
    Over and over I talked about living life, engaging with others, being part of the world. It is easy to say, and in many moments, almost impossible to live by.
    I will never say that life was easy, that cancer was easy, but I will say that I have learned more in this time that I have in the last 10 years of my life. Paying attention to my own feelings and heart gave

me the gift of insight into a world that I would never had known unless I was diagnosed with cancer. Cancer was a gift, and one that I will not take for granted.

I do not know where this life will take me, or how much time I have left. But none of us have that knowledge; we are all living on borrowed time. What we choose to do with that time is up to us.

How are you going to use your time?

www.ingramcontent.com/pod-product-compliance
Lightning Source LLC
La Vergne TN
LVHW011937070526
838202LV00054B/4688